Growing Sophia

The Story of a Premature Birth

Rochelle Barsuhn

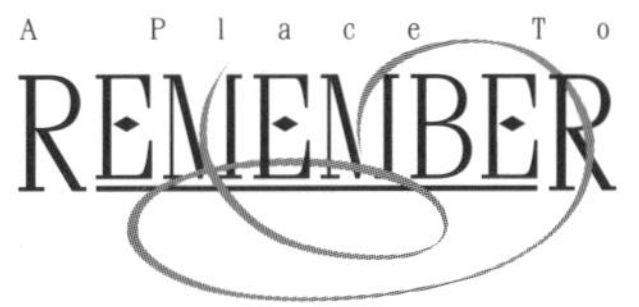

A Place To Remember
A subsidiary of deRuyter-Nelson Publications, Inc.
Saint Paul, Minnesota

Book design by Scott Barsuhn

Publication Data
Barsuhn, Rochelle D.
Growing Sophia: The Story of a Premature Birth
Includes biographical references
ISBN 0-9650848-2-5
1) Premature birth - Personal narratives.
2) Premature birth - Case studies.
3) Premature infants - Care and treatment - Personal narratives.
4) Parents of premature infants - Personal narratives.
5) Parents of premature infants - Psychological aspects and coping.

Printed in the United States of America
deRuyter-Nelson Publications, Inc.
1885 University Avenue, Suite 110
Saint Paul, Minnesota 55104

Acknowledgements
The author wishes to thank the many individuals who contributed to the nurturing of this book: Bruce Ferrara, M.D., Jean London, L.I.C.S.W., Lori Vandersteen, R.N., and Kathy Werner, R.N.C., N.N.P., P.N.P. for bringing to the review of book drafts the kindness and generosity they brought to the care of Sophia and her parents during their stay at Children's Health Care, Minneapolis; Sarah Nairn, R.N., M.S.N., I.B.C.L.C. (Children's Health Care, Minneapolis) and Jolene Pearson, Parent Educator (Early Childhood Family Education, Minneapolis Public Schools) for sharing their usual plethora of good ideas in the resources listings; Calvin deRuyter and Timothy Nelson for envisioning a need for this book; L.B. Norton who isn't so jaded after all of her editing projects that she doesn't still cry over manuscripts; Barb Trostad-Peterson for volunteer proofreading on short notice; Scott Barsuhn for living through this experience with me, and for reliving it in this book; and little Sophia for reacquainting me with miracles.

For the nurses

It takes more time to gestate a premature baby—or any baby in crisis—than a full-term infant. When there's no break from pain, time slows. It's like being in labor. The contractions keep coming, never giving you a chance to catch your breath.

During our daughter Sophia's hospitalization, tender people said to us, "You're so brave. I couldn't do it." But we weren't brave. None of us were. We would have taken the coward's way out in an instant. We coveted relief, a simple solution. Though we sobbed and railed and gave up more than once, we recognized that there was no escape from this. We had to go through it.

Sophia showed the way by struggling to survive, as very ill people do, in silence. We sat beside her, doing what was for us also instinctive—struggling with her.

Before

Why on this morning do we decide to take pictures?

As July sunlight floods the dining room, my husband and I finish a roll of film. First I photograph him sitting on a chair against the wall. Our dogs, two Yorkshire terriers, are perched on the chair beside him, leaning forward as if anticipating a treat. They are illuminated. Scott is in shadow.

Then I sit at the dining room table, my back to the light. My face has "the pregnancy puff" I had hoped to avoid, but I am smiling with oblivious happiness. Light wreathes my head. I have fed this pregnancy quantities of milk. I have walked three miles around Lake Harriet each morning. I am thirty-five years old and should settle down and take on a maturity befitting motherhood, but I am too giddy with the joy of gestation. What doesn't show in the photograph is the slight roundness of my abdomen, "the cantaloupe," as Scott and I have begun to call it. I am nearly twenty-four weeks into the pregnancy, ready to begin my third trimester.

The cramps began yesterday afternoon. They are so faint, so gentle, I believe they are growing pains. My brain tells me I'm not worried even while I skip the usual morning walk. Scott and I don't talk about it. In the car, we are in good moods. We are only driving to work—to the graphic design studio we own and that owns us.

There is the usual banter among employees over coffee, then we disband to our work. Normally I am steeped in projects, but earlier in the week I cleared my desk of oppressive deadlines. I feel unusually free. Still, it isn't until mid-morning that, as a precaution, I call the medical office and am surprised when the certified nurse-midwife on duty says, "I think we should see you."

I park the car outside the medical building and feed the meter only enough change to cover an hour of parking—just long enough to be assured that this is nothing serious.

The office assistant is kind and solicitous, but strangely sober. She tightens the elastic fetal monitor strap around my abdomen and leaves, closing the door behind her. The air conditioning cools the white-painted room. The machine clicks, emitting paper tape that shows seismic rises and falls. A red, heart-shaped light on the panel blinks rhythmically—the baby's heart is strong.

The midwife enters, looks at the tape, and tells me I am in labor.

When I learn I am being admitted to the hospital, I am incredulous—and embarrassed and self-conscious as the office assistant pushes me in a wheelchair through the skyway to the connecting hospital's labor and delivery ward. There is a holdup with the room. A cubicle is found in recovery. I get up on the gurney, and the nurse pulls the privacy curtain. I lie back, refusing offers of a hospital gown. I'm not sick. The labor will stop, and I will go home. We have dinner plans tonight.

The nurse secures a fetal monitor strap again and starts an IV of magnesium sulfate, a drug used to stop early labor. I am given an injection of betamethasone, which I dimly understand will help to mature the baby's lungs. Scott arrives. He sits inside the cubicle with me. There is hardly room for us, with all the machinery. We don't talk much. Scott is an unusually competent person who can be temporarily undone by calamity. He assumes the worst, and sometimes believes he is not strong enough to face disaster. We're both thinking about the baby and—what seems more frightening at the moment—the work waiting for us back at the studio. We have worked together at the design firm since the beginning of our marriage, and we both know what even a short-term absence by one partner will mean to future workloads and deadlines.

Now I am experiencing the full-blown side effects of the drug—hot flashes, nausea, the shakes, double vision. A new patient is pushed into the room, a woman still unconscious after a cesarean section. Her husband captures the moment by videotaping her lying on the gurney and by making calls to family members to announce the birth of a six-pound, four-ounce girl. This cannot be real.

The midwife reappears. "I've brought Dr. Olson," she says, introducing the perinatologist from the office. "He can tell you a little about what's ahead." The doctor tells me I can expect to spend the rest of the pregnancy—four months—in bed. Our plans collapse around us.

That evening after Scott, weary and serious, has gone home for the night, the contractions finally stop.

Labor

I am awakened by a nurse who has come to take the latest round of blood pressure and temperature readings. It is one a.m. She whispers, respectful of my sleep, lighting her tasks with only a flashlight. I drowse.

Then slowly I sit up, leaning against one elbow. Even in the dark I know what is wrong. "I'm bleeding," I call out, as I might have cried to my mother, with fear and the hope that she can make it all right. The overhead light flashes on, and I see the bright blood on the sheet, the gown, my legs. Panting with fear, I'm remembering last summer's miscarriage, the blood on the white bathroom tile. "It's over," my brain says clearly.

The midwife is summoned, along with the resident on call. Ultrasound equipment is wheeled into the room. Blinking, I try to focus on the slippery gray shapes the resident points out on the screen—the head, an arm, the spine. "The placenta is low-lying," she says. "Possible abruption. It's pulling away from the uterine wall."

I dial the phone, dreading the moment Scott picks up. I, at least, am cared for. He is alone. "I'm sorry," I say when he answers. "I'm bleeding. The labor has started again." There is no protecting him. I picture him putting on the jeans he just draped over the bedroom chair, going to the garage in a daze, driving past houses no longer lit with warm light.

In her gentle way, the midwife tells me I am being transferred to a hospital specializing in high-risk deliveries. She is grave but says, "A twenty-four-week fetus can withstand a lot of blood loss," giving me hope.

Three emergency medical technicians arrive and swaddle me for the transport across town. Scott comes in, fear on his face, in time to repack my clothing and drive it to the new hospital.

The back of the ambulance is lit as brightly as a living room. The EMTs make friendly conversation. I smile, I converse, I answer questions, floating above this nightmare. One of them tells me, this being a point in common, that his wife is twenty weeks pregnant. I imagine her at home in darkness, lying on her left side which is, the books say, the correct position to increase circulation to the baby. It is the position I slept in last night, pillows propped comfortably around me. I envy her.

The no-nonsense nurses who meet us in my new hospital room are equipped for an emergency. In minutes they have me cleaned up, in bed, and hooked to an IV bag of magnesium sulfate, a medication I have already learned to respect for its potent effects. Again, the crisis subsides. The drugs work. The contractions stop. Scott falls into exhausted unconsciousness on a fold-out cot next to my bed. I spend twenty-four hours lying in bed nauseated, shaking, and blinking with double vision. After the euphoric pregnancy, this helplessness is humiliating and shocking. I collapse in the arms of the nurses whose task it is to help me up to use the commode.

But when I am gradually weaned from the Mag—already I am conversant in the lingo of this new world—I begin to feel better. By Sunday I feel wonderful, even a little guilty for taking up a hospital bed. Friends stop by with flowers, piles of magazines, and candy, which is beginning to look delicious again. Scott smuggles in the dogs, who lie next to me on my clean hospital sheets.

That night, I am deemed stable and moved to a semi-private room on another floor. My medication is changed to oral terbutaline. Even with the tightness it brings to my chest, and my racing heart rate, it is a victory. No more IV.

Scott goes home. A nurse comes in and rubs my back, something I will owe her for the rest of my life. I sleep, finally.

When I wake, it is the middle of the night. The lights are out, the privacy curtain is stretched around my bed. I am lonely. Hospital lonely. My uncomfortable roommate, pregnant with thirty-week twin girls, tosses and shifts, watching TV and huffing behind the curtain. I earlier discovered that the volume control on my television is broken, so I can't rely on it for solace.

Again I fall asleep—deeply at first, then fitfully. When I wake again, it is early morning. I find I am still in the hospital bed. My roommate is still watching TV. I stuff pillows behind my back. My abdomen feels taut and alarmingly tender.

When the contractions return late morning, they are so intertwined with the general discomfort I have been feeling for the past several hours that I don't, at first, recognize them as labor. The fetal monitor has no trouble identifying them. The magnesium sulfate IV is restarted in a rush. A silent nurse sits on my bed making notes on a chart for what seems like hours, while the fetal monitor records sharp rises and falls on the white ticker tape. I have to breathe hard and concentrate through these contractions. Even as they grow stronger, I refuse to believe this is serious. Prayers, faith, patience, good behavior, bedrest, and the wise perinatal staff at the hospital will stop the labor. If all else fails, the drugs will work their magic, like aspirin on a headache.

The afternoon blares on. The waves of pain roll over and over me. Once more, I have to make a call to Scott at the office. "Please come—" What a failure I am, what a weakling. I stare at the red blink of the baby's heartbeat for reassurance.

When the backrub nurse—a woman who had been unfailingly cheerful the day before—comes on duty, I ask, just to be certain, "You're going to stop the contractions, aren't you?"

Her answer makes my heart dip. "We're trying," she says, her eyes avoiding mine.

Birth

I am lying on my side on the delivery table. Another contraction begins to take hold. It starts as pressure, grasping my abdomen as if this will be a gentle touch, a comforting one. But it tightens, squeezing, until it is high, sustained pain. I breathe in and out, afraid to panic, willing myself to go limp. Slowly the contraction subsides, and I descend from a faraway place.

The baby is coming. Only after being wheeled under a sign reading "Labor and Delivery" have I come to believe it is inevitable. My last hope, the magnesium sulfate IV, has been discontinued.

The room is filled with strangers. Two labor nurses. A perinatologist. A neonatologist. Two nurses from the newborn intensive care unit. I am overwhelmed, outnumbered, but my panic is submerged by drugs and the rhythmic pains. I lie on the table without protest. Labor is paring my senses to a necessary few. When the pain of each contraction subsides, hearing is the sense most acute. Someone suggests that Scott change into scrubs. Periodically one of the OB nurses calls out the state of my cervix like a football score.

"Six centimeters."

"Eight centimeters."

The temperature in the room is over ninety degrees so the baby, who has not yet built up fat stores, won't lose critical body heat when it arrives. Scott fans me with a clipboard, his expression grim. The contractions are for me a brief escape from the bright sterility of the room and the knowledge that our child—the one who is so real to us now, already so much a part of us—may not survive. Scott has no escape.

The neonatal nurse practitioner from the newborn intensive care unit—NICU—of the children's hospital next door has already given it to us straight. "A twenty-four week fetus probably has a fifty-fifty chance of survival. We'll reassess once we see it." Clutching a clipboard, she had been all business. The lungs were the biggest concern. At this gestational age, a baby wouldn't be producing enough surfactant, the lubricating substance that coats the alveoli, or lungs' air sacs, and prevents the membranes from sticking together. With the baby's first breath, the lungs would collapse.

Then she held out hope. A relatively new synthetic surfactant replacement could help. The baby would most likely need to be placed on a ventilator for life support. Once "intubated," it would be transported to the NICU. There was a myriad of possible complications—heart and lung problems, a potentially life-threatening intestinal infection called necrotizing entercolitis, the high possibility of brain hemorrhaging, which could result in cerebral palsy or mental retardation. . . . There were a lot of machines and monitors and drugs that might be used. Were we interested in hearing about them now or, did we want to wait until later?

"Later," I say, trying to be polite, but having a hard time appearing interested through the contractions. Only one fact makes sense to me; the baby has a fifty-fifty chance. This seems like a note of hope. At the last hospital the perinatologist told me babies of twenty-four weeks gestation had only a two percent survival rate. Did I hear wrong?

Doesn't matter. My mind is turning off now. My body is consuming all my energy. The nurse gives me a ten-second primer on how to push.

I feel a rush of warm amniotic fluid. This is it, I think, the last moment the baby is inside, safe, and for a moment I don't tell. I'm afraid. Then I say quietly, "My water broke," and all hell breaks loose as everyone rushes to get into sudden position. Another contraction, and I feel the baby's head coming. The perinatologist is without his gloves, and while he gets them on, the nurse helps me breathe against the immense, surprising urge to *push*.

With the next contraction I take a breath and push, once, but not hard, afraid the baby will fly across the room.

A girl.

She is born crying. Her cries sound artificial and high-pitched, like a baby doll's, but they are forceful. The doctor places her for a moment on my abdomen to clamp and cut the umbilical cord.

My vision returns in a rush, with relief, elation. She is clean and beautiful. I am surprised how beautiful. She is startlingly small, a baby in miniature. Her hair is wet and dark, pasted to a head no bigger than a tennis ball. Her arms and legs are waving vigorously. She is as thin as an old man.

"Poor baby," I say, sorry for her, cupping her head in my hand. Her eyes are fused shut like a kitten's.

Then the neonatologist comes and with gloved hands takes her to the warming table. The NICU team leans over her. Her crying stops abruptly when they thread the ventilator tube into her throat.

"Do you have a name picked out yet?" asks one of the OB nurses.

"Sophia," I say. It is the name we had planned to keep secret four more months.

Reality

The attending neonatologist invites Scott to accompany the team to the neonatal intensive care unit of the adjoining children's hospital. Later Scott tells me this was a difficult moment for him, deciding which patient—his wife or his new daughter—to accompany. But the doctor's invitation is not so much an offer as an address: "Dad, come with us."

In the months after Sophia's birth we will review every detail of this day, so I can picture the team descending in the elevator, pushing the plastic transporter unit on wheels. One of the nurses "bags" the baby as they roll through the hospital basement, squeezing the rubber bulb of a hand-operated ventilator with her gloved hand. Sophia's fragile bird chest puffs with oxygen.

Automatic doors open. They pass through an angled corridor that runs the length of two city blocks. It is hot, overheated by metal ducts. At the end of the corridor, more glass doors swing open, and they pass into the basement of the hospital. They ride an elevator up two floors and enter the NICU, a stronghold of beeping monitors, plastic incubators, and personnel in blue scrubs.

Scott stands back as a team of nurses gathers around the unit. He watches as they transfer the squirming red infant to an isolette, insert the IVs, attach the monitors, position the bright phototherapy light for warmth. Then the neonatologist who was present at the birth invites him into a private conference room for The Talk.

In it, he fills in the details left out by the NICU nurse in the labor room. There is no good news. There are additional complications not earlier mentioned. There is a strong chance Sophia won't live through the night.

"We'll call you if anything changes," he promises, as if in reassurance.

Afterward

I am taken to recovery, where I feel strangely euphoric. The nurse gives me 7-Up, and friends who have been called at the onset of the emergency are allowed into the room. They enter hesitantly, their faces a confusion of emotions—*should we be happy or sad?* Hugs. Jokes. My exhilaration unbalances them a bit. I am overjoyed. The baby is alive.

Monica puts a small box in my hand. "I want you to have this." Inside is a tiny gold lapel pin, a guardian angel. "I wore this before Maggie was born."

I am touched by the gift. Tim and Monica have lost several pregnancies and a baby stillborn at eight months. The last child, Maggie, is a miracle—a child said during prenatal ultrasounds to have severe physical defects, but who came out perfect.

"You don't know what will happen," Monica says, "so enjoy every minute you have with Sophia now. Then, no matter what happens, you'll always have wonderful memories of her." It is terrible to hear. It is, perhaps, the wisest advice I will receive during Sophia's hospitalization —a call to readiness, reality.

Scott returns to the recovery room, looking as if he has been kicked in the stomach.

Our friends disperse, and the nurse pushes me on the gurney to the NICU to see the baby. A flock of NICU nurses in blue scrubs part as we enter and stand at a respectful distance. One of them has already filled out a cheerful birth announcement. It hangs on the wall, declaring in neat, pink letters Sophia's name, birthweight—one pound, seven ounces—and the date, July eleventh. Our names appear beside the "proud parents" entry. This is the hospital staff's small gift to us, the carrying on of normal birth rituals.

I stare through the plexiglass of the incubator. After the birth high, numbness has set in, dumb and buzzing. Under the glare of the warming light, our baby looks like a tiny space alien. Her head is oversized and her arms and legs seem, for lack of baby fat, elongated and thin. She looks like one of the extra-terrestrials in *Close Encounters of the Third Kind*. Her eyes are shrouded in gauze to protect them from the light. There are plastic-coated wires running in tangles from adhesive patches on her skin to the machines outside, tracking her heartbeat, respiration, blood pressure. A catheter has been inserted into her bloody umbilicus.

Perhaps to give us a memory of physical connection in case our daughter doesn't live, one of the nurses encourages us to open the porthole and touch Sophia.

Hesitantly—out of curiosity and not for any comfort it gives either me or her—I place my finger against her tiny foot. The baby jerks. I feel strange and detached. I am relieved when the labor nurse offers to push me back to the maternity ward.

I am returned to my room. Scott goes in search of food. An OB nurse comes in for my blood pressure reading and to massage my abdomen. She can hardly find my incredible, shrinking uterus. Once she leaves, the room is very still. If it weren't for the IV pole I am tethered to, I could imagine myself in a hotel. The quiet, in fact, makes me think of arriving at our hotel room after our wedding reception—how, when Scott and I closed the door, the din and excitement ceased, and it was just us and ringing silence. I am in a daze of exhaustion. "Please, God." I am on my knees, clutching the IV pole. "Let her live."

It is late. Scott returns and, still in the scrubs he wore in the delivery room, lies down on the fold-out bed across the room. I get into my bed. "It doesn't matter which side I lie on now," I think, closing my eyes, expecting to fall instantly into dreams. But I remain floating on top of sleep, hallucinating. In the dark we both lie motionless, terrified that the phone will ring.

Changes

So we have a place of rest—the room where my insurance company says I may stay for forty-eight hours. When daylight of the next morning comes, we see that it is a festive place. The walls are painted a soft mauve. Balloons and bouquets festoon the other rooms, and visitors come in joyful surges to visit the parents of full-term babies. I don't feel this as a deep hurt. It helps, in fact, to be on the outskirts of the celebration, to recognize a fact that at moments escapes us: "Yes, you had a baby."

Scott pushes me, gallantly, in a wheelchair along the long corridor to the children's hospital.

We meet more neonatologists.

We establish the beginnings of relationships with Sophia's nurses.

We learn the foreign tongue of the NICU: Sats. Desats. Blood gases.

We look to the monitors, with their glowing red or

pulsating green readings, for truth and mercy.

We watch our daughter's chest. It inflates and collapses and inflates again with the unfaltering rhythm of the ventilator.

And gradually we understand that everything about our lives has changed. Until Sophia's birth, our days centered around certainties we did not question. The importance of our work. A healthy respect for clients and their deadlines. The need for food and rest. Now these things don't matter. We function well, but we are stunned, as if we have emerged from an explosion. Our ears are still ringing and the debris is filtering through the air around us.

By the day of checkout the seriousness of our situation has sunk in. No flowers have arrived. No one has come to visit. And although the OB nurses ask to see our one Polaroid photograph—taken by a sensitive NICU nurse on the day of birth—I recognize that they are being kind. Our baby, bright red, her face hidden by ventilator tubing, holds up one minute, skeletal hand as if pleading, "No."

Then, just before checkout, a bouquet arrives from friends, with an enclosure card: "Congratulations!" It gives us sustenance awhile longer. We keep moving.

We spend the day at the NICU, not leaving for home until exhaustion drives us out, well past dark. It is hot, midsummer, and the windows are rolled down. I have the sickening sense that we are driving away from our baby. During our crisis the world has continued. The crowds are out in shorts and sandals, on their way to restaurants with friends. The air sounds of laughter and traffic. It smells of barbecue. Everything seems lush and jewelry-bright. My eyes, already accustomed to the fluorescent lights and beeping machinery of the hospital, struggle to adjust.

The terrible loneliness doesn't begin until we reach the garage and carry my bags to the house. The garden seems overgrown. The morning glories bloom hysterically. I was so many months from expecting a birth, having a baby in my arms isn't what I miss; it's the pregnancy. I feel empty and no longer magical. I stand behind Scott as he unlocks the door, and I don't think I can face it, this site of our former life. The door opens and the Yorkies surge out, leaping around our feet. They seem huge, and the joyous barking of Keist, the outspoken one, seems misguided.

Then we see that friends have filled the kitchen with the day's arrival of bouquets and presents. A helium "It's a Girl!" balloon sways on a ribbon. I read the cards with a feeling like relief. Again, our achievement has been recognized—we have a child. I need these reminders.

We field incoming calls from anxious family members. Call the NICU for a heartening positive report by Sophia's night nurse. Struggle with a rented breast pump that knows more than we do. It is hours before we get into bed.

The book on my nightstand is a week-by-week guide to pregnancy loaned to me by a neighbor. It says a baby born at twenty-four weeks has virtually no chance of survival. We have already been warned about publications with copyright dates even a year old—the field of neonatology is advancing that swiftly—but I can't help taking this as ominous news.

We lie on our backs, side by side. It has only been days—eons ago—since I nudged Scott and said, "Look at that! The baby is moving again!" Sophia is no longer with us.

Sophia

The pink antibacterial soap is perfumed, deceptively sweet. We lather our hands and arms and rinse—then, superstitiously, lather and rinse again. After just a couple of days in the NICU we know a few grim facts. A simple cold virus passed to our infant could lead to her death.

Though I am drawn to them, I don't look at any of the other babies as we move through the aisle of isolettes. I fix my eyes on Sophia's incubator. Hers is the only misery I have stamina to face. I feel brittle. One light tap could send me hurtling in pieces, like shattered china. Somewhere I read that the reason newborns like to be swaddled, the reason they stop crying when they are held tightly—even too tightly—is that they have an innate, instinctive fear of flying apart. That's how I feel now. I have the sensation that my limbs are only loosely attached, that they could fly away. The social worker, an understanding woman with luminous eyes and the dramatic dark hair of Jacqueline Kennedy, compliments me. "You appear to be doing so well."

Sophia is having a bad day. In the delivery room she had been vigorous with outrage. Now, she sprawls almost motionless on the sheepskin fluff. She's losing weight. Her skin is wrinkled and flaky. Every so often she jerks violently. The nurse says that's normal—a sign of her unfinished nervous system.

We can't depend on our daughter to breathe. She's having apnea spells—periods where she stops breathing. The monitors blink their peaceful red digital readouts, then suddenly alarm. The nurse amazes us with her calm response. She touches a button to silence the buzzer, then stands observing the baby. Still no breath. She opens a porthole and wiggles Sophia's leg. At last, our daughter resumes breathing. Seeing that the oxygen saturation level in Sophia's blood has dropped, the nurse bumps up the concentration of oxygen flowing through the ventilator and stands watching until the machine says the level has climbed back into the nineties. Our nerves are jangling, but the nurse appears not to be unnerved by this event. "The parts of Sophia's brain that control her respiration are still immature," she says. "She'll outgrow this." Then she turns and records the incident in Sophia's chart. Everything is chronicled—input, output, medications, and subjective, detailed observations.

The nurse is our key to understanding, perhaps to surviving. She knows what all the machines are for, but more important, she can look at our baby and read *her* signs—something we don't know how to do yet. She is one of six primary nurses and a host of others who will contribute to our daughter's twenty-four-hour-a-day care. In the level three nursery the ratio of nurses to babies in Sophia's fragile condition is one-to-one.

We hover, asking questions. I have to be careful not to push too hard, because I want to know everything she knows, *now*. It is with relief and amazement that I find she is generous with her knowledge, and patient. There are no secrets. While she monitors and makes notes, she talks. We struggle to catch the terms she drops. Hematocrit. Bradycardia. Ampicillin. This is learning by immersion.

Light and the high commotion of technology swirl around us. The air smells of chemicals. I sit on a high, wheeled stool and gaze at the baby. There is a delicacy to her, a scaled-down perfection that is stunning. Her features are minute. Her hands, especially, are lovely. They move with the grace of a ballerina. Her hair has dried to a brilliant metallic copper; it grows in a perfect swirl at the back of her head. One of the nurses in the unit confides, "Oh, I don't like those big, fat, full-term babies. I like these cute little ones."

I stare at my daughter, separated from her by plastic, a formidable barrier. Touch is one of the first deprivations of premature birth.

Grief

My body is going back to normal. Before the first week is up I am back in my old clothes. I wash the hardly worn maternity clothes and put them away. The voluminous brocade dress my mother sewed for me. The giant new nightgown. I didn't even get to wear them.

In the half-darkened NICU, Sophia lies in her isolette looking alone. What does she miss? The powerful sound of my heartbeat? Warm amniotic fluid? The spongy parameters of the uterus? She comes from a space that had walls, a top, and a bottom. Now she flounders in open space. A nurse has taped the cone of a tiny diaper around her legs "so she'll feel her boundaries." I wish I could return her to that comfort, for both of us.

I am not ready for this pregnancy to be over. My brain and my body remember too vividly being happily fat with her. I felt good—round and productive. The grief I feel now is more than disappointment. It is deep loss.

Where I do most of my mourning is in the pump room. The hospital staff has been diligent in offering breast pumping instruction and equipment to the sudden mothers of preterm babies. Though very premature infants are not yet supposed to be passing milk through their digestive tracts, there is evidence that they process breast milk better than formula. Mothers can freeze their pumped milk in the large NICU freezer for the nurses to thaw as needed. I have taken up the challenge.

Every three hours I hook myself up to the ridiculous breast pump. I am tricking my body into thinking it is making food for a baby of enormous appetite and a perfect sucking rhythm. The pump exerts an excess of energy for its task. I am no match for the machine. There are dried splatters of milk in the mesh of the pump room chair. Dolly Parton smiles at me from the cover of a discarded women's magazine.

Though I am religious about this routine, no milk is coming. The plastic bottle attached to the plastic cones attached to the plastic tubing attached to the bovine pump is, after twenty minutes of vigorous suction, dry. I sit and cry to the puffing cadence of the machine—for Sophia who is suffering and for my own unfathomable sadness. Tears splash on my bare chest.

I press the suction cones against my breasts with one arm and write furiously with my free hand, listing what I miss about the pregnancy, the things I was just beginning to enjoy:

Having the baby with me.
Getting rounder.
Reading about labor and delivery.
Anticipating October.
Wondering what body part is developing this week.
Thinking about buying bigger bras.

Drinking decaffeinated coffee.

Dreaming of a baby party.

Asking questions during prenatal visits.

Drinking my milk.

Holding my stomach.

Outgrowing my pajamas.

Allowing myself coffee-chocolate malts.

Planning the birth.

Then, suddenly, days into the pumping, I see the first bubbles of wetness in the cones. The milk is starting. It is a soft color like melted French vanilla ice cream. It doesn't overflow the sterile plastic cups provided by the NICU, but it warrants a place in the big hospital deep freeze. I am impressed with myself. The pumping doesn't change the injury my dreams have suffered, but it gives me hope.

Once started, the milk comes in with a vengeance. In the middle of the night I have to page a nurse midwife for help, any relief. She talks me through what turns out to be engorgement. The term, as painful as it sounds, comes nowhere near describing the true agony of the affliction it describes. I find myself on all fours, soaking in the bathtub at three a.m. There appears to be no end to the humiliations.

Pumping gives rhythm to the days. I can only get so involved in activities before I must go pump again. My leaky body demands it. Feeding the pump is like feeding a baby—a new, purposeful obligation.

Lungs

In the x-ray, Sophia's delicate shoulder and arm bones look like pinned wings. The neonatologist points to the computer screen, showing me where fluid is collecting in the baby's lungs. The condition is called pulmonary edema, and it may be causing her sudden need for increased ventilator support. The picture of Sophia's chest reminds me of an aerial view of complicated waterways now swollen and overflowing their banks. He is starting her on Lasix, a diuretic to help her excrete the excess fluid.

I nod. "Anything," I say, "whatever will help," knowing that no treatment offered here comes without a price; this is an environment built on Catch-22s. The condition from which she suffers, respiratory distress syndrome, requires that she be placed on a ventilator. But the ventilator causes chronic lung disease because it damages the tissue in her lungs. The only encouraging news is that though the scarring is permanent, Sophia will eventually grow healthy new lung tissue. It is a distant promise. In the meantime, our task is to pray fervently that Sophia will be one of the few babies of her gestational age and weight to escape more serious complications; the NICU staff's job is to keep her breathing.

Every three hours a respiratory therapist—RT—arrives to administer a nebulizer treatment. While Scott and I watch, she rumbles Sophia's chest with a powerful vibrator, then holds a tube filled with vaporized medication to Sophia's face. Her objective is to loosen congestion in the lungs. The treatments seem rough, but Sophia doesn't fight them much any more. The more invasions she endures the more she seems to resign herself. We are all resigning ourselves.

Now the RT disconnects the endotracheal tube from the ventilator and rapidly inserts a suctioning tube into her trachea. If the ventilator hasn't been silenced ahead of time, it sets off an alarm. Of all the warning signals we hear in the NICU, this is the most frightening, for it announces that Sophia's link with air, with life, has been detached. The RT uses the tube like a vacuum. It sounds like a dentist's hose. It isn't until the vent tubing is hooked back up that we realize we've been holding our breath.

Affection

This is our daughter, we are her parents, but we feel like visitors to a stranger. I still call her "The Baby."

We have titles, too. Some of the nurses and doctors refer to us as "Mom" and "Dad," pseudonyms at once familiar and strangely distant, as if learning our names, when the outcome is so chancy, is not a good use of time.

I know the nurses are looking for signs of bonding. After each shift they note in Sophia's chart any contact with the family and whether we have asked questions or appeared affectionate with the baby.

Scott has no trouble expressing his emotions. Immediately. He hugs the isolette. He calls, "I love you, Sophia," when we leave the NICU.

I am shy with her. I feel self-conscious telling her I love her even though I have begun to feel sudden, strong emotions toward her. The feeling of connection surprises me, almost bowls me over. Before her birth, I had sincere doubts that I could muster up the necessary maternal skills to be anyone's mother. I didn't believe in instinct. But now bonded seems an inaccurate term, a description of superficial skin-to-skin attachment, like glue. This is more powerful. It's only been a few days, but I have fallen for her.

I begin two journals.

One is for Sophia. It records the highlights of her treatments, her doctors' pronouncements, her tiny achievements. ("You wrapped your hand around the ventilator tubing today.") I address each entry to her, beginning it with a schmaltzy endearment. "Cupcake . . . Lamb . . . Angel . . . " It is out of character for me, and I don't know her well enough yet to take the liberty. But the names are a way to express the frustrated need to mother this baby, an honest reflection of my tender emotions for her.

The other journal is for me. It is full of grief and margin notes and misspellings and crossed-out words. I am grateful for a place to try to think straight, but I don't so much figure anything out as rant and sob. There is such an onslaught of information coming at us, I must trust my hand to record what I know my overloaded brain will not. With so much downtime in the NICU, time spent just sitting and waiting, writing in the journals gives me a faint feeling of productivity. It may be the only worthwhile thing I am doing.

I have by simply and patiently watching her come to *know* Sophia. She has a personality. Likes. Dislikes. Familiar gestures. She chews or sucks on the endotracheal tube. She rests her arm on her belly or throws it back over her head. I see her rolling her eyes—maybe trying to open them. Her movements make me lonesome for her inside. We were just getting to know each other.

The scent of baby powder makes normal mothers think of their infants. It's the smells of the NICU—the hot plastic scent of the isolette, the citrus fragrance of adhesive remover, the unidentifiable chemical odor that clings to the breath of the nurses and our clothes—that I associate with Sophia.

Work

I am taking a few weeks off. Though I am stopping in at the studio to do sporadic work, I spend most of my time with Sophia. Scott says he can concentrate knowing one of us is at the hospital with her.

He has, almost immediately, returned to work. The choice is made for him—by the demands of the studio, by our financial obligations, by project deadlines, by responsibilities to employees. But we both know even if he could spend all day every day at the hospital, he wouldn't. He can't. Though he is overwhelmed by the workload he is shouldering, he feels best doing normal chores. He has to stay connected to real life.

Sometimes I bring work from the office to the nursery. One afternoon I try to write ads for a client. I sit in a rocker by the isolette and work, straining, for hours. Nothing gels. There are no sparks. I don't make even minor progress. My brain has turned off.

Stimuli

A preterm baby is not a small full-term baby.

It is a simple and profound truth I unwillingly acknowledge during an informational parents' meeting at the hospital soon after Sophia's birth.

The parent educator at this gathering, who is here to gently initiate us into the world of prematurity, shows us a video about the signals of premature babies. These infants have emerged months early from a muffled, dark environment and are easily overwhelmed by noise, light, even mild sensory stimulation. We learn that normal parenting behaviors—touching, talking, singing—may be inappropriate.

All of this information is tempered by the fact that parental involvement is good for the baby—even essential. But it needs to be modified to fit the premature baby's special needs. Only one stimulation at a time—eye contact, but no talking. Talking, but no touching.

To identify when the stimulus is too intense, we can watch for signs of stress.

Averted eyes.

A change in skin color.

Grimacing.

A drop in heart rate.

Apnea spells.

In the brochure provided I recognize one of Sophia's gestures—hands in front of her face, shielding herself, a pitiful and ineffective barrier against the invasive and necessary procedures of the NICU.

Raw-edged and frayed, we are overstimulated too. Noise, television, even books are too much. I stop listening to music. The CDs I had enjoyed the week before Sophia's birth are returned to the library. We avoid the parents' lounge, which is always crowded and where game shows play loudly on the television.

The pump room is, at least, private. Now while I pump, I just sit, exhausted, or—if I have the energy—scan magazines. I've read them all already, but since I don't have the concentration for real reading any more, it doesn't matter. The articles about baby-raising seem remote, so I skim the ones about pregnancy and labor. "How to Recognize the Warning Signs of Early Labor . . . "

Patience

After we park the car in the ramp and take an elevator to the connecting skyway, we must walk two long hallways to the neonatal intensive care unit. As we complete the first hall and turn down the second, our pace quickens. Now we are almost running, but I feel as if I am wading through a swamp, hardly moving at all. For four months, reaching the doors to the nursery is the longest portion of our journey to see Sophia.

Time has changed. Days disappear, with no accomplishments crossed off our list of obligations. We weather bradycardia and infection. While Sophia's doctors and nurses counter anemia with blood transfusions, and apnea spells with medications, we sit next to the isolette waiting for this to end. In this way, each day—while being completely unpredictable—is exactly the same as the one before.

I want to see progress . . . growth . . . success.

Weight gain is the easiest and most tangible proof of headway, and we track it religiously. But even that fluctuates erratically. One day she's up an ounce; the next she's down an ounce, plus an additional fifteen grams.

It has dawned on me how much waiting is ahead. Patience will be needed, more patience than I possess. Some days we see improvement. Sophia's ventilator pressure can be lowered. She has fewer oxygen saturation drops—incidents when the percentage of oxygen in her blood dips to a dangerous level. We leave the hospital feeling good. Then, when we call for an update a few hours later we hear that she has had several bad spells since we left.

Because I suddenly have time for such things, I chart the days on a graph. I subdivide the graph top to bottom and number the sections one through ten. Each day I plot my mood. A low falls near the bottom of the graph; a high hovers near the top. The chart shows wild rises and falls. What it doesn't show is that sometimes there are ups and downs even within one day.

My moods don't always mirror Sophia's current condition. I arrive one morning for another day of waiting, and the nurse greets me with a good report. Sophia is doing fine. I nod and take my usual place beside the isolette. I slump down, fighting for composure, feeling desperate, lonely, and frightened amid the bustle of the nursery. Trying to keep from sobbing in public is an ongoing agony.

Guilt

I spend futile time wishing I could take back the week before Sophia's birth. My brain obsesses over the events leading to her arrival. Did I take too many long walks around Lake Harriet? Could I have gone to see the midwife sooner? Could I have, with greater caution, kept her inside, floating in weightlessness?

Sometimes a wave of rational thought follows: "You did all you could. You went to the hospital. You took the medications. You would have stayed in bed for four more months. Maybe the bleeding would eventually have killed Sophia. 'Sometimes it's better for these little ones to come out,' that's what the perinatologist said in the delivery room. You have to believe everything turned out for the best." Still, I keep reliving that weekend before her birth, wishing for the power to go back and redo everything. As if I had ever been in control of this ride.

Two weeks after the birth, my parents and Scott's

mother arrive on flights from out of town. It is a relief to finally celebrate Sophia's arrival with someone. We stand around the isolette in a hush of awe at her smallness. Sophia, who has already shown herself to be full of surprises, presents us with a small accomplishment. We return from lunch to find a sliver of dark showing under one eyelid. Her eyes are opening.

After the first excitement, a powerful wave of sadness hits me. Needles, plastic tubing, strangers in scrubs. Her first sight of the world is of the NICU, and I am to blame.

Risks

A week after Sophia's birth, we have our first "care conference." It is our chance to meet with one of Sophia's physicians and other primary care givers in rare privacy and an unhurried atmosphere. We can ask our many questions and hear the doctor describe our daughter's condition. The nurses tell us we can request a conference any time we like. The staff's concern for us still surprises me. I remember the stories of my parents standing outside the hospital nursery after my twin brother and I arrived seven weeks early. During the length of our hospitalization they got no closer to us or our incubators than the glass in the nursery window.

No meeting rooms are available, so we follow the neonatologist and social worker into the on-call sleeping quarters. We sit on the bed, the social worker stands, and the doctor perches on the edge of the desk and tells us in rapid detail the potential hardships ahead.

The complication we fear most is the brain bleed. The pressure applied to Sophia's head during delivery or changes in her blood pressure could cause the fragile-walled blood vessels in her brain to rupture and bleed into her brain tissue. This hemorrhaging, the doctor tells us, most often appears within the first few days of life, and in severe cases can result in mental retardation, cerebral palsy, and physical disabilities. There will be three ultrasounds of her brain—one today, another at a month of age, and a final one just before she is discharged from the hospital.

By now I am so exhausted that I can sit tearless and ask questions without my voice quaking. Scott, overwhelmed by information, grows serious and quiet, sitting with hunched shoulders next to me.

A few days later, as I am passing through the central lobby to Sophia's room, the neonatologist on duty puts his caller on hold to tell me, "Head ultrasound came back normal."

I turn and go back through the doors to the parents' lounge where Scott is sitting drinking coffee. His head is bowed over the cup, and I move toward him, smiling. I am carrying good news and our first moment of real happiness since our arrival at the NICU.

Differences

There is a separate crisis going on. Scott and I are trying hard to support each other, but our relationship is pulling at the seams. The stress intoxicates us, exaggerating our worst traits. As our differences come out, we are by turns loving with each other and angry beyond reason.

At the hospital, Scott is Mr. Gregarious, everyone's friend. The nurses love to see him coming because he jokes, laughs, puts everyone at ease. On even the tensest days he talks loudly to Sophia and calls good-bye to everyone when we leave.

The stress of the NICU just heightens my usual inwardness. When I come into the nursery I feel systems closing down. I have to know, "How's Sophia?" before I can relax and chat. I crave quiet.

The low-frequency tension between us erupts more and more often.

He accuses me of being cold to the nurses. "You could try harder."

I accuse him of insensitivity, of putting his social life ahead of his daughter's welfare. "We don't have to be best friends with the world," I say. "Sophia is more important than being bosom buddies with everyone in the NICU!"

"I do need to be best friends with the people who are taking care of my baby!" he shouts.

Inane. We have no problems with Sophia's doctors or nurses. But this isn't about logic. Neither of us is ready to recognize that we are both coping as best we can.

Our differences become the most difficult part of Sophia's hospitalization, at least for me. I am confused by my husband's outgoing social behavior when at home he seems silent, angry, depressed, and pessimistic. He fantasizes about escape. "I wish we were getting on a plane for a two-week vacation." "I wish I could just spend the day on a lounge chair in the back yard." He says that he wakes up each morning and is hit by everything in a rush: "This is your life." Much as he loves Sophia, he hates the hospital. Although he visits every day, he has a dread of spending long periods there. He has no good memories of the nursery and thinks only of the trauma of care conferences, IVs, and transfusions.

I view this, with great pain, as disloyalty to Sophia. I don't want escape. As horrible as time at the hospital sometimes is, I want to spend every moment there. It makes all the other stresses in our lives—work, finances, our relationship—for a time, vague. I wake each morning thinking of Sophia, and the hope of getting to the nursery soon is what pulls me out of bed.

One of the nurses, now also serving as confidante, theorizes that in this crisis men take on too much of the burden and responsibility. Scott is at a disadvantage. Not only is he dealing with the daily traumas of our business, he hadn't experienced the high of birth and the attachment that comes with (an albeit short) gestation.

Scott and I try, awkwardly, to give each other room.

I spend many hours at the hospital while work piles up. I cram cleaning and shopping into Saturday mornings, then race to the nursery.

Scott gets busy with home projects, the ones scheduled for completion before Sophia was born. House painting is the most arduous and pressing of his tasks, and now that the window molding has been removed, it must be completed by fall. He pushes himself without mercy. On the hottest days of the summer he heat-strips old paint off the woodwork.

After an afternoon of necessary but exhausting errands, I come home to find Scott collapsed on the couch. He's been working outside since early morning. His forehead is sunburned. His eyes are closed. I put down my grocery bags and stretch out with him, pressing my cheek to his chest. I hear the beat of his strong heart. We don't say anything. We just lie there, gripping each other.

Hope

The old neonatal intensive care unit, the nurses tell us—the one the staff moved out of a few years ago—was a big open room lined with incubators. It was noisy, more like a big warehouse filled with equipment than a nursery.

There is no disguising that this new space is a high tech environment, but the architects have *tried*. The unit is divided into separate rooms branching off a central reception/work area where the social worker, charge nurse, and doctors sit answering their phones and doing dictation. We share space with five other isolettes and two private chambers used for the treatment of babies with infectious diseases. There is a cheerful wallpaper border of ducks marching around the perimeter of the room.

Although Sophia's room is lit only by artificial light, there are windows in the room across from us. Occasionally, after a day under fluorescent lights, Scott or I will suddenly look up and see sunlight through those windows. It is always a surprise, a reminder of good, simple things we have forgotten.

We cling to bits of encouragement offered by the nurses.

"She has good skin."

"She comforts herself well."

"I just have a good feeling about Sophia."

These are as close to guarantees as we can come in this place.

Despite the ups and downs, even while I worry and suffer, I have an illogical belief that she will do well. This isn't Pollyanna optimism; it is confidence mitigated with realism. I know we may see some horror before this journey is over.

Puzzled because I am not usually an optimist, I mention this to a former college professor. She says with quick, deep surety, "That's a gift from God."

Exhaustion

Weariness moves in and dries us like a hot wind. I feel parched and dusty—and look it.

After four weeks of part-time work at the office, I have returned to a full-time schedule. By 5:30 each morning, we're up. Scott can't sleep any longer, and I have a dire need to pump milk from my hard and leaking breasts. One of us calls the hospital for an update. Did Sophia have a good night? Any spells? Did she gain weight?

While I pump, Scott leaves for a several-mile bike ride around a string of city lakes. Though he is under no less stress and has borne the bulk of the studio burden, he looks great—tan and trim. He reminds me of himself when we were first married. A week before Sophia's birth, after getting a surprisingly high cholesterol reading, he put himself on a low-fat diet. Now he tracks his vegetable, fruit, and saturated fat intake with fervor, carrying a chart in his personal calendar. It is satisfying to have control over this small portion of life.

With the pumping done, equipment washed, and the bottle labeled and stored, I shower. Scott returns. He showers. We drive to work with briefcases, dogs, and our new mascot, the ubiquitous breast pump.

At the studio the phone rings incessantly. There has been no let up in the pace. I sit and look at my computer monitor. Things don't make sense to me. Nothing seems important. I write an enthusiastic proposal for a project and think, "I'm just playacting."

I ache with loneliness for Sophia. I call the nursery at intervals, desperate for any information, frustrated by the brief updates. In the meantime, there's work to be done. I am inundated with obligations and depressed at my ineptitude at meeting them. The copywriting projects are too much—heavy and entangling. Too many options. I don't want to think creatively. The most I can handle is concrete tasks—make this call, add this column of figures. The chaotic day is interrupted by pump breaks every three hours. The studio freezer is filling with small plastic jars.

We have to move fast during our brief energy spurts.

By the end of the day, we're almost sick with exhaustion. One night we go for dinner to get our energy up—Nikki's restaurant for salads and pasta. We sit at the counter by the window so we don't have to stare at each other. The food fills us up but doesn't make us any more energetic. While waiting for the bill we try to use our time wisely, plotting out the weekend, who will do what. It boggles my mind. We have to go over details again and again before they make sense to me.

At the hospital, we gaze at Sophia and, when invited, help with her "cares," as the nurses call them, turning the verb into a noun.

We change her diaper, swab her dry mouth with sterile water, and report her temperature so it can be logged on the chart.

We read the nurses' reports and the doctor's orders.

I inevitably make a trip to the pump room.

We say good-bye.

It takes a long time.

Then there's the drive home. Each night the mundane tasks that lie between me and bed seem insurmountable. More pumping. More equipment washing. Bottle labeling and storage.

Then, for a brief time, we sleep.

Dreams

Sleep becomes a favorite hiding place. We don't expect rejuvenation; we just look forward to temporary unconsciousness.

Each night, I have every parent's anxiety dream. I dream that I must save my baby. She is missing, and I have to get her back into her safe hospital bed. Or her wires have been disconnected and the monitor lost. One night I dream that Sophia is caught under ice in a lake. I dig her out with my bare hands. She is gasping and cold, but still alive. The circumstances of my dreams change, but the theme is the same.

Scott gets used to being awakened by my frantic searching in the bedding.

"Sophia's not here," he says calmly. "She's at the hospital."

At first I am confused.

Then I am irritated, thinking he is the crazy one.

Finally, I am relieved. I sink back into my pillow. For the time being, the baby is safe.

I have never been responsible for anyone else's safety, and I'm not doing a very good job of protecting Sophia. I am, in fact, doing nothing to shield her from the treatments and procedures of the NICU. It panics me, and I attempt to quell my panic by sitting beside her incubator with my scrubbed hand through the porthole. I can hold her whole hand between my thumb and index finger. Her fingers are limp but warm. Then I can breathe. I am doing something. I am holding onto her.

Success Stories

Before Sophia's birth, I hardly realized babies born prematurely were at risk, and I didn't know many people who had given birth to a preterm infant.

Now former premies are everywhere. They come forward in a crush. They are all grown up, and doing just fine.

Everyone we have ever met was a premie. Or knows someone who was. Or had a cousin, an aunt, a grandmother who had one. It is a funny cliché among NICU parents that everyone has a great uncle Ollie who was born weighing two-pounds-something and miraculously survived when his parents tucked him into a shoebox and kept him warm in a coal-burning oven. I'd laugh, but our family legend involves great-grandfather Albert Jipson and his twin brother Arthur, born in 1882. The doctor estimated their weight at two pounds apiece and said they'd never live, but the parents, being German and bullheaded, wrapped them in cotton batting anyway, put them in shoeboxes, and kept them in the warming oven of the drafty farmhouse's coal-burning stove. To everyone's surprise, the babies got fat. They grew up, took up farming, and lived into their eighties.

So people tell us their miracle stories, as if these foretell a happy outcome to our crisis. So many premature babies have done well for themselves. Not only did they live and thrive, but they are doctors, writers, adventurers, fathers, mothers, composers, Ph.D.s! The only ones who don't tell us success stories are the doctors. They offer statistics, instead. If, after a week, Sophia is still alive, her chances of having a life-threatening "incident" will decrease. Only half the babies Sophia's age and weight experience bleeding in the brain. . . .

Almost no one tells us stories about premature babies who have cerebral palsy or who didn't make it, but we know about them. Through the privacy panels carried in for the occasion we hear a doctor preparing a couple to make a decision about their ventilator-dependent baby who has suffered a serious brain hemorrhage and will always be disabled. Amid tubing and equipment we glimpse the gnarled, contracted hands of a baby with a severe brain injury. We hear a nurse softly asking the parents of a baby who is dying, "Would you prefer that I call a priest or a chaplain?"

In this environment, it is difficult to envision that other people's successes have anything to do with us. Hooked to IVs and monitors, Sophia looks sick. She looks as if she may die.

She reminds me of the baby starling I found last June, the month before her birth. Its mother had built a nest on top of a concrete overpass near our office, and it had fallen into the parking lot below. It lay with its skeletal wings sprawled and tufts of downy feathers poking through its raw-looking skin. It tried, pitifully, to hop away from me. I put it in a cardboard box and Scott drove at breakneck speed to the refuge center run by the University where volunteers attempt to nurse injured and abandoned wildlife back to health. I haven't heard, yet, whether the bird survived, but I know from experience that even when you do everything right for a bird that falls too soon from the nest—keep it warm, feed it, and lock the cat out of the room—it most often dies.

One day, Sophia's nurse comes into the unit, smiling. "There's someone here you have to meet." She leads me to the lobby where a mother waits with her little boy. "This was a twenty-three-and-a-half weeker," she says. "He was one sick baby." She shakes her head, as amazed as anyone at his recovery. He is over a year old now, and very active. He climbs on the stroller, looking out of place here, where the babies lie prone and vulnerable.

The nurse is pleased, glad to have shown me *hope*. But as I sit again beside Sophia's incubator, I can't imagine what this story has to do with me. I am happy that things turned out all right for this baby, but Sophia is still in crisis. The nurse and the graduate mother see what I can't—an end to this. It seems I have always sat beside this isolette. It seems that I always will.

Postpartum

My postpartum check-up comes during what should have been my twenty-ninth week. I make my appointment with the nurse-midwife who admitted me to the hospital.

There are two other women in the waiting area when I arrive, each cradling a new baby. As I sign in, they are swapping names and admiring the dark hair, plump cheeks, and beautiful wise eyes of each other's infants. They are obviously strangers to one another, but have the instant and intimate rapport of women who have survived labor and are now rapturously in love with their babies. I take a seat, holding my photo album on my lap. I can't wait to get out of here. Their cheerfulness is killing me.

The office assistant calls me back to the examining room. I haven't seen the nurse-midwife since the night of my transfer to the hospital, and I'm anxious to speak with her. She is connected with a happy past when I was pregnant, and now she is connected with Sophia.

When she comes into the examining room, we hug. We share memories of the same ordeal.

I have a lot of questions. Mostly—*why?* There are possible explanations for the early labor—the perinatologist had recommended a dye study at a future date to determine if my uterus is misshapen—but no answers. That's something I'm going to have to live with.

I show my pictures, which she examines with the proper gravity and admiration. I tell her about the emergencies Sophia has overcome since her birth, and what dangers are ahead. I am prepared and controlled. I don't break down in the telling of the difficult parts of the story.

We say good-bye, and I go out to the car. I feel calm for the rest of the afternoon, detached, almost tranquilized. I have gotten good at holding myself back.

Pasta

Eating has become an imposition—something we must do and which takes time away from Sophia—so we skip meals or spend only the time it takes to walk to the hospital cafeteria. The vegetarian selections in cafeterias are less than extensive, so we eat multitudes of cheese sandwiches. I can hardly eat fast enough. I can't wait to get back to the nursery. Scott and I are both losing weight.

Then, by accident, we discover something that gives shape to the week. Pasta.

Every Saturday night I attempt to amend seven days of trauma with a dinner of fettuccine in red sauce, or spaghettini with black beans, cilantro, sweet corn, and tomatoes. I make whatever strikes me. I don't read any recipes. The fragrance of garlic cooking in oil fills the kitchen. Bits of parsley fly. The pasta dinner becomes the one dependable event in an unstable week.

We sit on the couch and drink wine. We feast on

huge platefuls of pasta and watch a rented video—anything that requires no intellect and no concentration, something stupid that we would have walked past with scorn in years previous.

This ritual brings something like pleasure back to our lives, at least once a week. This time is sacred. We don't answer the phone. We don't, until the movie is over and the dishwasher is humming monotonously, talk about Sophia. Bolstered by fats and carbohydrates we lock up the house and go to the garage to make our late Saturday night trip to the hospital.

As hard as it is for me to be away from Sophia on these evenings, it is good to conjure the ghosts of yesterday's comforts. We can't pretend that the NICU doesn't exist, but we can for a moment admit that this sweetness exists, too.

Family and Friends

Visitors to the NICU are, literally, numbered.

We may choose four people to visit Sophia in the unit, and their names are listed on the official card posted beside the incubator. This policy is to limit babies' risk of exposure to infection and, I expect, to regulate chaos in an already hectic hospital environment.

Our card lists my parents and Scott's mother. Because they all live out of state, their visits will be infrequent. The final line remains blank. We can't decide whom among our local family and friends to choose. It becomes a huge dilemma for us, and we make no choice. The line remains empty.

It is a difficult thing, not being able to share the birth of a baby.

To soften this and other hardships, family and friends begin overwhelming us with kindness. While the doctors and nurses labor over Sophia, they come bringing their gifts. Flowers. Food. Loaned baby equipment (for the optimistic future). Breakfast. Plush toys. Mylar balloons to tie to the isolette. They pray for us. They call, asking for details about Sophia.

My sanity is saved by those calls, for I have an insatiable need to *tell*. Anyone who will listen hears the day's details, and there are always plenty. Scott says he is too exhausted just surviving each day's crises to have energy left over for retelling them. But we share awe and gratitude for the generosity of our friends and their interest in our daughter.

We are trying not to be bitter about the people who don't call or who make no attempt to understand—the ones who minimize Sophia's premature birth and seem to believe that a preterm infant simply gets put into a warm box to grow. Who can blame them? I romanticized my own early birth. My brother and I weighed just over four pounds apiece, and our smallness was legendary.

An acquaintance from my past stops by the studio, a fellow writer from another lifetime, when writing seemed important.

"What have you been working on lately?" he asks, giving me a lead-in.

Relieved that the topic has come up, I hastily bring up Sophia and the hospital.

"Oh, I heard you had a baby. How's she doing?"

I am just beginning the telling when he interrupts to discuss what really interests him, the beautiful paint colors in the office. "How did you ever choose them?"

On the opposite side are people who treat Sophia's birth as a potential tragedy, who say offhandedly, "I didn't want to give you a gift for fear she wouldn't make it."

We decide to have our first dinner with friends. The nurses are enthusiastic about this. They think it will do us good. People are always telling us, "Go out! Have a good time!" I am ambivalent about this advice, appreciative of the concern, but surprised by the naiveté. Do they actually believe we can enjoy a carefree evening? During a telephone update one day, a nurse—she is a kind woman, but she hits me wrong this time—says, "You know, you don't have to spend every moment here. We'll understand if you take time off to do other things." I hang up the phone, weep, and then write in rage, "My baby is in intensive care! I want to be with her! Will everyone stop telling me to go to the movies!"

But we know there is wisdom in the idea of taking a break. We'll try it. Maybe they're right.

We meet our friends at a restaurant we once called our favorite. Almost immediately we recognize this outing as a mistake. Our fault. We are too deeply embedded in crisis to be good dinner companions, and we're not strong enough, yet, to deflect bad news. Three of their friends have had premature babies—two babies now dead and one blind from retinopathy of prematurity, a risk Sophia now faces. The meal is interminable. We have lost our ability to eat a leisurely dinner.

Mostly people are gentle with us, as if we are still gestating, as if they are afraid to disturb a delicate pregnancy. Our family members call daily. Friends, wary of being pests, check in every few days.

We finally add Sandy's name to our visitors list. She is the logical choice, a sensitive soul, a woman who has weathered a birth crisis of her own. During a routine ultrasound a little over a year ago, she and her husband, Chip, were told that their baby had hydrocephalus. Since then the baby has been born. She has had surgery to insert a shunt and shows no signs of problems. She is a perfect child, beautiful. Sandy knows uncertainty and endurance.

We meet her at the NICU one Saturday, nearly seven weeks after Sophia's birth, and wait for her to scrub up. She looks scared as she enters the unit and comes toward the incubator. She leans over and looks at Sophia through the plexiglass. She is silent. Then she says what we didn't realize until this moment we were desperate to hear.

"Oh, my gosh, she looks just like you guys!"

Bad Advice

"Just forget about this place."

"See a movie."

"Go out to dinner—just the two of you—and don't talk about Sophia or the NICU."

"Take a drive somewhere over the weekend."

"Go back to work. You can't do anything here."

"Sleep in tomorrow."

"Stop worrying so much."

"Don't get excited about the highs, and don't get depressed about the lows."

"Don't worry about the monitor alarms."

"Have another baby."

"Why don't you step into the parents' lounge while we do this procedure?"

Pain

The doctor has ordered an IV for insulin to counter skyrocketing glucose levels.

"You might want to step outside while I insert the IV," says one of Sophia's primary nurses.

"I'd like to stay," I tell her.

"Are you sure?" she asks, genuinely concerned. "This won't be fun."

There are a million things I could do—go for a walk, stop in the gift shop, make calls from the parents' lounge. But being away makes me feel disloyal and cowardly. More and more I feel a need to hover, watch over. It is a protective urge. Scott calls it my "she-dog" instinct. "Remember how Keist was about her puppies?" I laugh in recognition. Then again, maybe instinct has nothing to do with this; maybe this is the only rational response to carrying a fetus inside for six months—feeling her kick, watching my body grow in response to her growth. I've decided I can't abandon Sophia just because it is difficult for me. Someone strong is needed to stand by her.

My job is to hold her head while the nurse searches for a vein. The procedure begins. The nurse feels Sophia's leg and then, at the designated spot, pushes the IV tubing through her skin, twisting to thread it into the vein. Sophia thrashes, but the ventilator tube silences any crying.

No luck. The nurse withdraws the IV, bandages the spot, and moves to Sophia's arm. Again, failure.

I am sweating. It takes all of my resolve to stand by and allow this to happen. The nurse, too, is frustrated. She tries the other arm. The vein eludes her. Another nurse is called in for assistance. The two nurses bend over the baby. I cup Sophia's warm head between my hands. There is nothing I can do for her, and my helplessness makes me want to sob.

When the IV is finally established in her hand, the nurses tape on a splint to keep Sophia from removing it. It is so heavy she can hardly move her arm. I step back, feeling weak.

Successes here are short-lived. That night, as I return to the nursery after a nine o'clock pumping, Scott comes toward me. "Her new IV's leaking," he says. Clearly, he wants to be the one to tell me, understanding how this will hit me. "They have to put in another one." The evening nurse is already feeling Sophia's arms.

"Why don't you two step out for a while?" she says, looking up. Her suggestion is weighted with authority. It makes me irrationally angry.

But Scott also is insistent, and I follow him outside to the central lobby. We stand around, getting in the nurses' way, hoping that the procedure will go quickly. Finally we go sit in the deserted parents' lounge. An old batch of coffee sits on the hot burner in a glass carafe, condensing to a deadly black. I pace. I don't know what is wrong with me. In the grand scheme of things, in the multitude of traumas Sophia faces, a new IV is a tiny matter. It isn't life or death. But I am unraveling.

Forty minutes later, when no one comes to get us, we go hesitantly back to the nursery. Sophia's arms and legs once again show the bloody marks of failed attempts. The IV is in her head, illuminated by the bright overhead task lights. Scott, I am amazed to see, is able to pick up the pieces once again. He laughs and jokes with the nurses. I am speechless, near tears. Angry at myself for leaving. Angry at the NICU. Angry at the nurses for doing their job, and at my husband for being more rational than I.

In an attempt to warm and calm Sophia, the nurse covers her with a miniature square blanket. It casts Sophia's tired face in a comforting shadow. She calms down. She clasps her hands together and falls asleep holding them near her mouth.

Touch

We spend a lot of time standing back and watching.

During the first frightening days, I observe the nurses from a distance and have no desire to touch Sophia. She isn't the sort of baby a parent instinctively wants to cradle, but that's not what's holding me back. I might dislodge wires. Overexcite her. Do something terribly wrong. After everything she has been through, it seems selfish to subject her even to gentle stroking. She should be rocking in amniotic fluid, out of sight and out of reach for months.

But this is a place where touch is unavoidable. The neonatologists thrust their hands into the isolette and flip her over out of a sound sleep. Her arms fly out. She looks like a spinning whirligig. And though the nurses try to minimize handling, there is no sparing her. Sophia's feet are scabbed from heel sticks, the blood tests that are used to monitor her blood gases. The skin on her cheeks is raw from the tape that holds her breathing tube in place. There are hands constantly in the isolette.

My father says, "You need to develop a method of touching her that is unlike anyone else's so she recognizes you."

Scott and I begin, tentatively, to help care for her.

It takes skill to change a diaper amid a web of monitor wires. This isn't even a diaper at all, but two narrow strips of cotton batting, one between her legs and the other wrapped around her waist to hold the first strip in place. Temperature-taking is a greatly loved routine because it requires holding a digital thermometer under her skinny arm for a long minute or more. The nurses are patient with us, though it takes us three times as long to accomplish simple tasks.

Gradually I discover the comfort of sitting with my hand curved around Sophia's head, holding her hand, or cocooning her whole body between my two cupped hands. I don't know if it's doing much for her—I'm still learning to read her signs—but it's saving me. Once I make it to the nursery I can hardly wash my hands fast enough. If Scott and I arrive together, there's a race to the sink to wash up.

One day a respiratory therapist tells me about being a patient in the hospital herself years before, in great pain. A nurse came into her room and said, "Haven't you been given anything for pain yet?" and placed a hand tenderly on either side of the RT's face.

"I'll never forget the *relief* of that touch. I can still feel it."

I tell her of my first night in the hospital when I was bleeding and scared because I thought I was losing the baby. The midwife, who was sitting on my bed waiting for the EMTs to arrive to transfer me to the other hospital, touched my leg—just a comforting "I'm here" gesture.

There was strength and healing power in that touch. It was what held me together that night.

The RT says, with simple awe, "I get chills hearing you tell that story."

When Sophia's respiratory treatment is complete, the therapist closes the porthole doors softly. I drag my chair to the other side of the isolette, the side Sophia is now facing. Very gently I cup my hand around her head.

Magic

One afternoon, almost a month after Sophia's birth, I arrive at the hospital just as the nurse is preparing to do the weekly isolette switch. "Do you want to hold her while I get the new incubator ready?" she asks.

She dresses Sophia in a knit cap, diminutive flannel shirt, diaper, and socks, then wraps her in two blankets. I sit in a rocker. The nurse places her, tubing and all, in my arms. I stare down at her, breathless at her proximity. I can feel her movements inside the blanket, but she's so light it's like holding cotton candy. Or air. I feel woozy.

I must be sitting very stiff and still, because the nurse laughs and nudges me. "Relax. Rock a little."

Woodenly, I rock. I speak in a voice so soft it is almost inaudible. Gradually her eyes open. She looks up at me, squinting as if the lights are glaring instead of subdued. One hand wobbles around her face. It lasts ten minutes. It is magic. It wipes us both out.

Walking

Scott and I incorporate walking into our survival.

We walk the long underground hallway to the adjoining hospital's cafeteria—not really for the food, but for air.

We walk to a fast food restaurant for yogurt cones.

We walk to a local shop for coffee.

We walk around Lake Harriet, getting nowhere.

The Pregnant

The world is full of oblivious pregnant women. I avoid them, but they are everywhere. Their smiles are serene, as if they have no worries, no premonitions.

A woman from church whose due date was the same as mine is getting bigger and rounder.

On the patio of a local coffee shop, Scott and I are surrounded by fat babies and gestating women. I see no connection between these children and Sophia, but the pregnant women look familiar to me. I gaze at them in bafflement and admiration. We hunch and slurp our coffee, feeling out of place and conspicuous.

A new neighbor comes to the door, collecting money for an upcoming block party. We shake hands. Thirty seconds into introductions she tells us that she is pregnant—due in February. After she leaves it takes only the space between the front door and the couch for me to break down.

Privacy

A fat medical record book sits on the shelf near the isolette: Sophia's chart, the book of her life. Many people contribute to this text—RTs, nurse practitioners, occupational therapists, nutritionists, neonatologists. There are pages of doctor's orders . . . lab results . . . records of medications administered. Most informative is the narrative account of the day, as noted by wise and observant nurses. Each shift, the story grows.

We are allowed to read from this text. It is not filtered for our intake. We must decipher the abbreviations, decode the handwriting, and ask for translation of the technobabble in the lab readings. Generosity with precious information is a gift given to us by the NICU staff. It greatly helps me to *know*.

It isn't until I discover at the back of the book photocopies of my OB history that I begin to think of the book as a symbol of the privacy we have lost since coming to the NICU. This loss is still new to us. Although by his outgoing manner Scott gives the illusion of being open, he is protective of his privacy—a trait he is having, by degrees, to abandon. The medical office has asked about our finances. The social worker has, with sensitive questions, unwittingly made us cry. One morning I come into the NICU to find a bored nurse, one I've never seen before, with the record book open on her lap, reading about my prenatal obstetrical visits.

The hospital is where we lose, if not our dignity, our modesty. Mothers come straight from the delivery room in bathrobes and hospital gowns. And because there is no private space for grief, parents do their breaking down in public. This, I have observed, occurs only after valiant efforts to remain in control. Though the strain of holding up and being brave is terrible agony, showing weakness is worse. Many times I ache to let loose the torrent of sobs caught in my chest. Sophia's nurse gives my arm a sympathetic squeeze, and asks softly, "Hard day?" Clenching my jaw to ward off tears, all I can manage is a nod. I fantasize about cry rooms, closets off the unit like phone booths—a place for parents to howl in isolation.

Because of proximity, it is impossible not to know which babies are in serious trouble. The parents of very ill babies look exhausted. Their nurses, too, contrary to the myth about professional distance, are easy to read.

Still, we all fight to maintain a semblance of privacy. There is an unwritten protocol here. We don't gawk at the other babies. We stick to our own space.

Visitors and newcomers to the NICU aren't always familiar with this convention. On one occasion I am stationed beside Sophia's isolette when a cheerful grandmother arrives to visit the full-term baby of her daughter. Sophia's isolette is draped with a quilted cover.

Not many years ago it was discovered that preterm infants gained more weight and recovered more quickly when they weren't left exposed in plexiglass boxes under harsh lights twenty-four hours a day. It's not as peaceful as the womb, I think, lifting a flap and looking at my sleeping infant, but it's an improvement. Under the cover, the light is muted, like sunlight through a canvas tent on a July afternoon.

The woman glances over at me and leans closer. "Is that a little premie in there?"

"Yes."

She reads from the birth announcement posted on the wall. "One pound, seven ounces. Oh, my. That's small. Mind if I take a peek?"

She lifts the corner of the isolette cover. This is just a brief trip to the midway for her. *See the freaky baby, two bucks.*

It is a constant struggle, searching out places of privacy. At lunch some days I can find an empty hospital hallway and eat in solitude.

One day, when Sophia is showing signs of improvement, I sit alone and eat a pasta salad. (It has finally occurred to me that the hospital cafeteria serves the world's unhealthiest food. Having grown tired of cheese sandwiches and having despaired of locating entrees that aren't deep fat fried, I bring a lunch.) Usually I eat quickly, without enjoyment, but Sophia has had a couple of good days in a row, no apnea spells, and today I eat with more pleasure than I have felt in weeks. I imagine us cruising through this hospitalization, right past the prophecies of trouble and the sober doctors' warnings not to get too excited about the successes. Our daughter is astonishing. When I return to the nursery I find that the baby across the aisle is in crisis.

He was born five days before Sophia, with a headful

of straight black hair. I know he has been fighting an infection—it's impossible not to know what's wrong with every baby in the unit, we are packed in that close—but I didn't know he was this sick. Five or six nurses are clustered around him. They are grim, intent on their work. The isolette is open, and the crash cart containing the equipment for emergency resuscitation has been pushed over. A male nurse is "bagging" him with a hand-held ventilator.

I hide beside Sophia's incubator, partially to escape, but also to give the baby a little privacy. Someone brings in a partition, fabric stretched over a jointed wooden frame. "Have the parents been called?" a nurse asks with urgency from behind the divider.

The family arrives, with a translator. They are Hmong and speak no English. How frightening it would be to be separated from information by language. Behind the partition, the baby dies. He is wrapped in a blanket. The family is escorted to the lounge for a few minutes to hold him in peace. The nurses disperse. The partition is taken away. The isolette is empty.

Within hours, a new premie arrives—"fresh baby," as the nurses call her—and we all resume our waiting, in public.

Calls

We telephone the hospital often—first thing in the morning, then at intervals throughout the day, trying to wait a reasonable period or for a shift change, as if calling too often is an embarrassing sign of weakness. I know that if I check in too much, I don't leave the nurse on duty any crucial information to communicate.

"I don't know what to tell you," says the nurse when I call an hour and a half after leaving the hospital for the evening. "Not much has changed."

She thinks I want *big* news—apnea spells, ten grams of weight gain, a blood transfusion. But what I crave is the nonessential information. Did she open her eyes after we left? stretch her leg? cry? wet? If she were at home I could see for myself that she fell asleep with her hands curled under her chin; I wouldn't have to pester anyone for this minutia. The details are what I miss.

The phone has become an important icon in our

lives. It rings constantly, linking us with grandparents, aunts and uncles, friends—all waiting the appropriate interval before calling again to ask, "Is she doing better? What happened today?"

Pictures

Because we have no photographs of Sophia's emergency delivery, we try to make up for it by taking rolls of photos during her first days in the NICU. These pictures will be the first evidence of Sophia that we can send to family members. We order four prints of each shot from the photo developer and plan the outing to pick them up as we would a first date.

The packets are fat and enticing, but we resist opening them until we sit down at the pizza shop next door. As we begin dividing the sets, we fall silent. In the photos, Sophia's skin is bright red. It has a grotesque, shiny smoothness. The gauze over her eyes is stark white. She looks like a burn victim. Why hadn't I seen this before? I try to keep the pictures from the gaze of the college kids at the next table.

We send the sets out to relatives with the following apologetic note: "Some of these are a bit gruesome. . . ."

Later, when I hear my mother-in-law has shown the photos to a friend, I lament sending them. The social worker says, "She *should* be proud to show pictures of her granddaughter." But it's not shame for Sophia that I feel. It's protectiveness. I want to shield her from the honest reactions of unprepared people. I am afraid they will look at her the way the insensitive grandmother at the next isolette did—as if Sophia were a sideshow. Thinking about this now, I wonder if perhaps Scott's mom looked at Sophia with the same oblivious love that had made those pictures such a surprise to me. Why would she expect her friend to be anything but admiring of her tiny new granddaughter?

But people do look at our photographs with horror. They can't help it. She is out of their realm of experience, and it takes an eye tuned to details to see her beauty.

During a driving trip, relatives make a special trip to Minneapolis. They are excited to see the baby, disappointed when we can't invite them into the NICU. Do we have pictures? Sitting in the hospital lounge, we pull out a few carefully chosen photographs. They are stunned into silence by the little, shriveled, old man, our newborn.

A client says the pictures don't bother him, he saw fetuses in jars at a state fair once.

A friend who saw Sophia in her incubator right after her birth admits, "I was surprised how much it upset me. I had to talk a lot about it afterward." My baby is traumatizing, like a car wreck. I understand, but I am hurt.

I don't know why I expect them all to look at her with love.

Even months into this, we don't recognize how far we still are from "normal." Toward the end of our hospitalization, when Sophia has finally grown plump cheeks from Decadron, a steroid for her lungs, a friend looking at the latest batch of pictures says with relief, "Oh, she looks like a regular baby now."

Extubation

Sophia grows impatient with the ventilator. The nurses find her tugging on the endotracheal tube and predict that she may extubate herself—take the tube out. One of the doctors who has a reputation for aggressive treatment has already suggested that it will soon be time to give her a try off of the ventilator. No matter how it happens, I half-dread it, imagining the horror of watching Sophia struggle for air—or worse, watching her be reintubated if she's not yet ready to manage breathing on her own.

She follows through one early morning six weeks after her birth—turns her head and pulls out the ET tube.

When we hear the news, we race to the hospital to *see*. For the first time since her birth, her whole face is visible—nose, mouth, cheeks. Only a tiny plastic cannula—flexible tubing with two prongs that fit into her nostrils to blow in oxygen—interrupts her features.

We don't even see it. To me, she looks exactly like my brother, Reg—all two pounds of her.

Another first since her delivery—we hear her. When we open the isolette portholes, her mews and the hamster-sized rattling in her airway sound above the rushing hiss of oxygen entering the isolette.

With the ventilator off, she can soon be transferred out of the NICU into the level two nursery next door. We have made tangible progress.

Moving

We pack Sophia's belongings, a whole cartload of essential stuffed toy animals, including the furry white elephant that plays "When You Wish Upon a Star" when the string in its trunk is pulled, making me weep. There is no doubt that the experience of Sophia's early birth has strengthened me, but it has also depleted my immunity to shameless sentiment.

We are leaving the place that Scott has called "a house of horrors." We are also leaving the nurses whom we have come to love and trust, and an environment that has become, if not comforting, familiar.

It takes a respiratory therapist and a team of nurses to wheel Sophia next door to her new home. The oxygen tank comes with us.

The level two nursery is quieter, darker. We are given space in a room that has a window and two other babies—one in an incubator, another in a crib. The nurses greet us as if we are friends. We meet the first of four new primary nurses. We unpack, apprehensively.

Sophia weathers the move without complaint. Her parents drive home, fatigued.

Separation

It's been a rough evening.

After several apnea and bradycardia spells—A & Bs, as we call them in the condensed jargon of the hospital nursery—Sophia has been turned to her back. She hates sleeping on her back. She is restless. A nurse has her radio tuned to a country-western station. The music adds to the surreal gloom. Another baby in the unit is crying, an awful cat-squawk cry.

A cloud of uneasiness has settled over me. An eye exam is scheduled for the morning. Sophia's eyes will be clamped open, one at a time, with a tiny metal device called a retractor. The device hangs in a plastic bag, like a threat, on the wall. I am trying not to think about it, but my mind pictures the nurse holding her immobilized in a blanket while the ophthalmologist pries her eye open with the retractor.

What the doctor is looking for is signs of retinopathy

of prematurity. It is a particular danger to extremely low birthweight babies, and Sophia shows signs of progression of the disease.

I have read and reread the brochure given to us by the nurses, memorizing the terms. There is a possibility that the blood vessels in her retina will continue to grow erratically, causing severe problems. If the condition advances she may need surgery. In the worst case scenario, the one we automatically jump to, she will go blind. Scott won't look at the brochure. It makes him angry even to talk about it. His defense against bad news is to know as little as possible about the risks we face.

He's working late at the studio, writing a syllabus for a class he will be teaching. In a few minutes he is coming by to see Sophia. Then we will drive home. Some evenings it seems unbelievable that we must *leave* her. Almost every night I shed surreptitious tears. Walking out the door is a huge leap of faith, an unnatural act. The better she does, the harder it becomes to walk away.

And though today has been a bad day, overall she is showing signs of improvement. Her arms and legs are pitifully thin and her knees are still wrinkled, but she's gaining weight. She's finally in clothes—a doll-sized T-shirt and a pre-premie diaper. I try to picture myself pushing her around the lake in a stroller, a simple wish that seems extravagant. Do other parents take this for granted?

Sophia is still writhing in the isolette when Scott comes in. He goes straight to the sink to wash up, and puts his hands through the portholes. He holds her fast, and speaks to her in a father's voice, tender and resonant. Sophia calms down and falls asleep. We have a moment of peace before the inevitable departure. When we get out to the car, I still have her scent on my hands.

The news we receive the next morning isn't good. The retinopathy has progressed. There will be another exam in a week. The waiting will continue.

Waiting is the only sure thing about our stay here.

Regret

On my disorderly desk at home I find a paper in my handwriting titled "Birth Plan," a hopeful document composed early in my pregnancy. When I read the list, I laugh. It was all planned out, this birth, like a studio project. I had done my research, read volumes of books, and had at long last come to an understanding with myself. This birth would not necessarily include medication, the usual interventions, or even a doctor. My plans were:

Stay at home as long as possible.

Wear my own clothes.

Up and walking.

No fetal monitors.

Subdued environment—low-lit, quiet.

Delayed cord clamping.

No separation from baby after birth.

Reality diverged from my plans.

In the delivery room, the perinatologist, upon

learning that I had planned to work with a midwife, quipped, "We'll give you a good midwife delivery." I wonder if he thinks he even came close. This is my memory:

No shortage of medications.

Down in bed.

Fetal monitors.

Bright delivery room lights, commotion, and don't forget the stirrups.

Doctor I have never met and nurses I will never see again.

Cord clamping in a hurry.

Immediate separation from baby after birth.

I was not even necessary. My uterus decided things and went ahead against my wishes. Medical technology handled the rest.

Though there are, even at this late date, pangs for the delivery I had planned, there is no one to blame. It takes time for my brain to accept that this was Sophia's birth, not mine.

I revise the list. This new one is short, but it outlines the important things, the reasons, big and small, for gratitude.

No episiotomy.

No cesarean.

Professionals in attendance.

Sophia made it.

Breastfeeding

Sophia gets her feedings by machine. Every three hours, a medfusion pump squeezes the contents of a syringe slowly through the naso-gastric tube that is taped to her cheek and runs down her esophagus. The nurses measure her meals in fractions of an ounce.

When one of Sophia's primary nurses suggests, after many weeks, that it may be time to start breastfeeding, we are pleased. Not only does it signify the reaching of a milestone, but Scott's shoulders are stooped and the walls are dented from hauling the breast pump and its big unwieldy blue plastic carrying case. For weeks it has traveled with us to and from the studio. We're a sight, staggering into the office building. We envision a future minus equipment. We envision a future of bringing Sophia home from the hospital.

The nurses warn that teaching a premie to eat—especially one born at twenty-four weeks—is a unique challenge. Apprehensive but determined, I only half believe them.

The clinical nurse specialist employed as a full-time lactation consultant meets me at Sophia's isolette. Behind the privacy curtain, she describes the breastfeeding process in simple terms. Packed in with pillows, supported by a foot rest, I awkwardly get the swaddled Sophia into a football hold. I lift her toward my breast, rub the nipple on her lower lip, and jump, startled, when Sophia opens her mouth wide and latches on.

Miraculous. Barely three pounds, and doing what she is programmed to do. I am dazzled by it. I am in love. I haven't felt like this since the moment after her birth. My daughter is capable of great feats. In the diminutive blue sleeper, Sophia rests in my arms, her hair a gorgeous copper. Work leaves my mind. This could go on all afternoon—it is very relaxing and purposeful—but it actually lasts about ten minutes. The lactation consultant congratulates us on our first attempt.

As Sophia's primary nurse hooks her up for the remainder of her feeding, the ominous pressures of work return, but I am in a new state of hope. Nothing can dilute this sweetness. Suddenly I'm thinking about life as a parent, projecting to a future. The pregnancy seems, at last, something past. The breastfeeding has worked a transformation. It reminds me of the moment when I first knew I wanted a child, a moment of clarity, like stepping into another room. Although the memory of my previous life—a place where I had been content—was still vivid, everything had changed, suddenly. There was no going back.

I am surprised that Scott is not as transfixed by this miracle as I am. He is solidly supportive of the breastfeeding, is even shocked by parents who decide against it, but he gets no joy sitting inside the curtain as I nurse Sophia. It is taking me awhile to understand how excluded he has felt during this whole hospital gestation. Though the hospital staff does its best to draw fathers in, this is a mother's game. He points out that there isn't even a space for the father's name on the isolette identification card. He takes this as a personal affront and challenge, and goes about exploding the stereotypes. He is a bit of an oddity in the nursery, not just involved, but hyper-involved—enthusiastic with the nurses and expressive with his daughter.

We discover, as predicted, that breastfeeding the premature infant is not for the weak of heart and resolve. Sophia isn't efficient at this new task, and I am merely persistent, not experienced. In our quest, the lactation consultant and I investigate every option. She suggests I try a supplementer system, a contraption designed, I think as I am trussed into it, for the purposes of humiliation. A canister like a plastic water canteen hangs by a thin cord around my neck. Two long, thin flexible tubes emerge from the nose of the canister. The ends of the tubes are taped to my breasts. The hope is that when Sophia is rewarded with gushing milk she will be encouraged to suck harder, longer. The lactation consultant has to stand beside me, clamping and unclamping the tubing to regulate the flow of milk. "Don't get discouraged," she says. "She'll probably grow into all this—she just needs time." Milk rolls luxuriously down Sophia's chin.

Practice. That's what's needed. I make early-morning treks, lunchtime treks, after-work treks. The sessions are, mostly, disappointing.

As usual, privacy is a rare commodity. Everyone from maintenance personnel to representatives of the insurance company barge into the room in the middle of breastfeeding sessions. A closed door around here must mean "come on in."

One Saturday morning Sophia suddenly latches on. Three hard pulls, five, eight, twelve. Then steady sucking and swallowing. I am afraid to move. It is lovely and amazing. There is a complex rhythm to this, a rippling like an anemone on an ocean floor. Victory. We're on our way.

At the next feeding she has forgotten everything she learned.

"Don't worry," say the nurses, joining the now familiar cant. "Don't get discouraged."

I'm not discouraged, just confused. Will it ever work? If Sophia figures this out, if she stops having apnea spells, we can spring the joint—give up the NG tubes, blood tests, and agonizing good-byes. She won't be released until she is taking all of her feedings by mouth and gaining weight. But we are standing still.

My body conspires against me. I am so keyed up by tension at the studio that even when Sophia sucks strongly for a minute or two, I am dry. I try relaxation techniques and visualization. Nothing. I don't let down until she has stopped sucking and started to fall asleep. She chokes on the sudden flow, dropping her heart rate and coughing. When I get her sitting up on the pillow, the look on her face is one of exhaustion and resignation.

We try an ad lib schedule—feeding on demand. I spend the night on a fold-out cot next to her crib, with baby blankets taped over the observation window. The hoped-for outcome: she'll get hungry enough to eat. I last through only one shift of Sophia's crying and frantic pushing away before I beg the nurse on duty to give her a feeding through the NG tube. The feeding tube is reinserted. Sophia coughs—hard—as it goes down, but she gets her meal.

We are both working very hard.

"I've never seen a twenty-four weeker take all her feedings by breast, and I've never seen a mom try harder to make it work," says one nurse to Scott.

During this period of great effort, Sophia loses weight. What should feel right and natural feels like a mistake. The doctor's dictation says that Sophia will probably need to go home on a milk supplement—HMF or human milk fortifier, a powder added to the breast milk. I read between the lines: "Mother's milk is inadequate. When baby breastfeeds she's not getting the calories she would get through the tube."

Weeks go by while I resist the nurses' offers to "bottle" Sophia, afraid it will confuse her when her breastfeeding skills are still erratic. One evening after a tense and frustrating day at the studio, Sophia is hungry when I arrive. She gets more upset with the delay of temperature-taking and diaper-changing. By the time I get rigged with the supplementer, she is in one of her hands-waving-fearful-face-covering spells. I'm so small-chested the neck cord of the supplementer has to practically strangle me to work. HMF and milk are leaking everywhere. I'm so tense I don't even let down. After twenty minutes of either jostling Sophia back awake or trying to calm the windmilling arms, I hoist her up and hold her against my chest (a difficult task with the supplementer around my neck). I am worn out. I was so confident that this would work out. It really was the last hope I had of giving Sophia a comfort and intimacy she has been missing since her birth. I call the nurse and tell her it's time to start Sophia on the bottle. Do I detect relief?

The bottle comes—thirty ccs of fortified milk. There is a brief discussion of the best nipple type. Whatever. Sophia has her bottle. She has it fast. The milk flows in.

I feel curiously weak, greatly disappointed. The nurse lets me give her a bottle with another ten ccs. It is an odd, bland experience after the intensity of breastfeeding. I'm not ready to give up the breastfeeding, not yet, but we're in limbo, and I feel like the big solid barrier to progress.

I leave Sophia in her crib to go pump and shed tears.

The nurses and I come up with a practical compromise. We will collaborate on a combined routine of bottle-feedings and breastfeeding. Anything to get this baby home.

Time

Everything takes too long—cleaning the house, driving to the work, getting a connection once I've dialed the number at the hospital nursery. I am in a perpetual state of anxiety. Scott and I have adapted to Sophia's slow progress. We know to applaud even minor progress as miraculous. But our patience with normal delays, leisurely pedestrians, and long lines is gone. Time has become too precious.

On a Saturday morning I wait for a prescription at the pharmacy. There is a holdup of an hour. Apologies and more holdups. I am breathless with tension. An hour out of my day! No time left to drive by the hospital for a quick visit, as planned. Instead I have to go home. I need to be productive, accomplish something, clean the house. But I feel awful. As I work, the tension that began that morning turns into a cramp in my neck. By late afternoon (I haven't even had the time to shower yet) I know I *need* to see Sophia. She's alone in that place, and I am certain it helps us both if I sit beside her for a time.

Scott says, "Go." A mercy.

After a brief visit, I feel better. I even have the enthusiasm to return home and cut up eggplant and garden beans for our weekend pasta dinner. We have our obligatory red wine.

Scott is euphoric: "I live for these dinners. I can handle the week if I know this is coming."

Graduation

When we arrive for a seven o'clock feeding one evening, a crib—pink sheets and all—is waiting in the wings. The isolette portholes are open. Sophia has been bundled in many layers since early afternoon—diaper, shirt, sleeper, hat, socks, two blankets. It's time, says her nurse, for the big move.

The crib looks like a cage for a wild animal. It is huge and gray, with heavy metal side bars. The nurse lets us remove Sophia from the isolette and place her on the mattress. We pack rolled blankets around her. She looks vulnerable, exposed to glaring lights, cool air, noise. We are suddenly aware of the hectic pace of the nursery. We have come to depend on the protective plastic cocoon. It is hard to leave her.

We adjust, as we do to all of the changes we encounter, but there are always new changes around the next corner. Our next change comes a week later.

"Another baby is coming over from NICU," says the nursery charge nurse, calling the office late one afternoon. "She needs to be in a 'big' room, and Sophia is stable enough now to move to one of our private rooms. Would it be all right if we transfer her?" She asks courteously, giving me a choice, and I say, "Yes, of course," thinking of the babies with serious problems we've seen in the past months. But when I hang up the phone there is a lump in my throat. Change? New nurses? Even after all the major stresses and serious worries, I still sweat the small stuff.

When we arrive that evening, Sophia has already been moved to the private room. She is lying in the big crib, looking around. She doesn't look stressed. Her black eyes are moving back and forth, assessing the new environment. She knows something is different.

Scott and I are less flexible. The room is noisy—noisier even than the big room in which we had started. It seems to amplify the commotion of the adjoining rooms. We feel anxious and disoriented.

Scott holds her while I straighten up the place. Then I turn off the overhead light and close the door. It is dark and cave-like in the room. It has only taken an evening; we are *into* the new private room.

Kangaroo Care

Scott and I have dinner together at a favorite old haunt. We need to eat, and we're trying to resurrect this old pleasure.

Scott seems depressed tonight. While we wait for our food (what's taking so long?), we try to converse about something important. We end up talking about Sophia, as we always do, and he shrugs, ambushing me. "I feel detached. I'm not important in the equation."

This is difficult to hear, when I feel so attached I imagine I have become a different person. I rush to reassure him. I tell him he *is* vital. I remind him of his ability to calm Sophia down with a touch or his voice. I can tell it's a futile effort. He nods, but he doesn't look any happier. We pay our bill and drive by rote to the hospital.

When we arrive at the nursery, the nurse opens Sophia's chart and in triumph points out new orders—

orders she has, no doubt, championed with the doctor: "Kangaroo care sessions twice per day."

From our early days in the NICU, kangaroo care has been held out as a jewel, a promise for the unimaginable future. During my compulsive reading I have learned that the practice began in 1979 in Bogota, Colombia. Hospitals with no access to incubators invited parents to hold their premature babies for hours at a time on their bare chests to warm them. Skeptical medical personnel were surprised to find that these babies not only survived, they thrived on the touch of their parents.

There is no shortage of incubators in the U.S. With such access to abundant technology, it has taken time for physicians to concede that kangaroo care is a positive, even beneficial thing. But resistance is wearing down. Since coming to the hospital I haven't met any doctors who are outspoken advocates of the practice, but neither have I met any who are opposed to it.

Scott is anxious to give it a try, can't wait to get his hands on the baby, in fact. He takes off his shirt and puts on an open-front hospital gown. The nurse undresses Sophia down to a diaper. She then removes her from the incubator and positions her on Scott's chest. The two of them are covered with a blanket. The baby is a tiny lump in pink knit cap. Her feet don't even reach to his waist. This is something new. She flutters her eyes up to see who's holding her. Then they both relax, as if under a spell. They're not asleep, but elsewhere, somewhere outside the hospital. Every few moments Sophia makes a noise I have never heard her make before, a contented, exhaled "Ahhhhhhhhh." When the session is over, the nurse practically has to peel Sophia's heated little body off of Scott's chest. She looks like one of those flattened cartoon characters who's been run over by a steamroller.

When we leave the hospital that night and walk the familiar bright hall to the parking ramp, Scott says, "I'm not detached."

Days later, when I am finally over a cold, I take a turn. I can't see Sophia's face—the only down side of this—so I have to go by feel. She is a small, solid pressure, very warm. Her scrabbly hands move a bit. I can feel her fingernails. Then she settles down and goes to sleep. I leak a little milk.

Kangaroo care helps us picture a future when she will come home. We imagine holding her for hours at a time, whenever we want. Though the nurses are indulgent and don't scrutinize their watches, there is a time limit to this bliss. We must always return her to her bed before we are ready.

Machines

Instead of being intimidated by machines, as we were early in Sophia's hospitalization, we now find them reassuring. Not only have we become used to them, we have grown dependent on them. The ventilator is gone, so we turn to the pulse oximeter.

We have special doctor orders—two kangaroo sessions per day, for ten minutes at a stretch. This is precious time, worth sums of money. We guard it and keep track of who went last. Occasionally, sensing a need, one of us will let the other hold her.

Sophia has so little energy reserve that even being held wears her out. When she gets tired, the numbers drop. The machines report any slipping of her heart rate or oxygen saturation level. They are like tattling big brothers. Just when we get comfortable, they tell, and a nurse has to hurry over and turn up the oxygen. After several sat drops she suggests, kindly, that it might be best to put Sophia back in the crib. Though we have been told that it is important for babies to be handled lovingly by their parents, we ascertain that our touch is dangerous.

I am the fortunate one holding her now, sitting in the big comfortable vinyl rocker the nurse has pulled next to the isolette. Sophia and I are alone. The privacy curtain shields us. Task lighting under the counter softens the darkness. It is far from quiet here. There is always pandemonium in a hospital nursery, always. Nurses talking, babies wailing, rustling garbage bags being replaced. But with Sophia in my arms, I am content. It surprises me how much I need to hold her.

I can't take my eyes off the monitor. Sure enough, the numbers begin dropping. I am silent, holding my breath as the oxygen saturation level slumps . . . 92 . . . 91 . . . 90 . . . hoping the numbers will rise on their own. 89 . . . 88 . . . 87 . . . When the machine reaches the preset danger level, it sounds the alarm. The nurse slips behind the curtain and turns up the oxygen.

We're not ready for weaning from machines yet. For the time being, it's us, our newborn, and high technology. But as Sophia grows bigger, our feelings about the machines are conflicting. They have helped to save our baby's life, but they are beginning to interfere with parenting.

Apnea

Though we are months into Sophia's hospitalization, the oxygen saturation drops and apnea spells continue. Sometimes we will have several good days in a row before Sophia has a series of events. She seems especially vulnerable during the evenings and early morning hours. When we call for a report after the night shift, we sometimes learn that she has had five or six incidents since we left the hospital the night before.

Then, as we near her due date, the spells become less frequent. One evening we come in and find the pulse oximeter sitting on the ledge, its electric cord dangling. The red digital numbers display is black.

It is replaced with an apnea monitor, which takes some getting used to because it doesn't have a continuous readout. We have to trust that it is working—that it will sound when and if Sophia stops breathing.

CPR

A pocket mirror—that is the practical gift given to us by the nurse officiating at the CPR classes we are invited to attend. Some premature babies have apnea spells even after they go home. They have a higher than average chance of dying of SIDS. The mirror is to hold under Sophia's nose when she is asleep to be sure she is still breathing.

The class is harder than we have imagined. Scott gets teary realizing that the doll on which he is practicing resuscitation could be Sophia. I feel myself going into Shut Down. It is a defense that I have perfected during weeks of hospitalization. We move through the A-B-Cs of CPR (Airway, Breathing, Circulation), and dutifully practice puffing breaths into our plastic dolls, thumping on their backs, and pressing two rhythmic beats into their chests to get their hearts pounding again.

Afterward we have an appointment with

representatives of the equipment company that will supply the apnea monitor coming home with Sophia. The two women take us into the parents' lounge and repeatedly demonstrate the piercing, almost unbearable, scream of the monitor. The alarm paralyzes me; I sit blinking while it shrills.

"Sophie," the women keep calling our baby. "How long has Sophie been in the hospital? When will Sophie be going home?" I'm frayed from months of tension, and this minor infraction hits me as a major irritation.

Then it is time to hook up the new monitor to get us used to it before it goes home with us. The hospital's space age video-screen monitor is turned off, and the electrodes attached to Sophia's skin need to be removed. They are affixed with strong adhesive patches. The two women move forward. They have performed this task before and bring practiced gentleness to their job, but as the adhesive begins to pull away, Sophia flails and cries with true heartbreak in her voice. Once again, there is nothing for us to do but stand by and allow it to happen.

Meltdown

The day begins falling apart during a morning meeting with a client. The budget is tight, and parameters keep constricting. All I want to do, now, is finish the project and be done with it. Today there is much waiting around, disorganization, and covering the exceedingly obvious. It isn't annoying so much as oppressive. I leave the client's office feeling weighed down.

I cheer myself up thinking maybe I have time to squeal up to the hospital for a moment. Scott and I share a vehicle, and I have to pick him up at the college where he is teaching a morning class—*his* current heavy burden—but if I hurry. . . .

Speeding, I get halfway there before I realize I'm not going to make it in time. I slow down, suddenly earthbound again. I drive back toward the college, park the car, and wait fifteen endless minutes for Scott's class to dismiss.

Back at the studio I work on one of several thousand hot deadlines while Scott races from appointment to appointment. A frustrating afternoon.

I call the nursery after lunch for my usual, much-anticipated check-in. The nurse gives me the perfunctory rundown, "Stable, lungs clear, tolerating feedings well. And," she adds, "Sophia is awake and looking around now." This information hits hard. The thought of her in bed alert and gazing at the ceiling while I am so far away working on meaningless projects makes me weak with despair.

I make a point of asking about the latest head ultrasound results. It is the last of the periodic ultrasounds scheduled for her, and we've been waiting to hear whether there are any signs of abnormality, any bleeding in the brain.

"The report is in, but hasn't been read yet," the nurse tells me.

"When will it be read?"

"Sometime late this afternoon."

I hang up feeling dissatisfied.

I postpone my next call until late afternoon. The lucky nurse to take my call is Sophia's primary. When I ask about the ultrasound, she hesitates. The report has been read, but there's something in the terminology that the doctor wants to question the radiologist about.

It is at this point that all of my worst fears come rushing in on me. I press for a time when this consultation will occur. No promises can be made. I get more aggressive. "We're going on our third day of not knowing the results," I say. I back off, then, suddenly remembering that I'm talking to our much-loved nurse, a woman who has always been on our side. "It's just very difficult. But if we have to wait, that's what we have to do."

After I hang up, I am shaking with—fear? No, anger. I call right back. "I have to have answers—tonight," I say, surprising the nurse with my intensity. "I don't care who talks to the radiologist; if the doctor's not available, somebody else has to do it." The nurse has sound, logical reasons why this may be impossible, but my sense of justice has been wounded, and I am not flexible. "I know the doctors see these things all the time . . . " I begin the sentence with calm authority, but halfway through it my voice quavers, and I finish, through tears, *"but this is our Baby Sophia."* The nurse assures me she will do whatever she can.

Scott is returning late to the office after a thirty-minute drive from a meeting across town. We have a dinner appointment with a friend in fifteen minutes. We collide in the downstairs hall of the office building, both of us ready to explode with our own frustration and fury. I rail at him, and he raves at me, and by the time we get back out to the car we are coming apart. He gets in the driver's seat and slams his door. I slam mine harder. The car rocks. We are both screaming. My voice is hoarse, louder than I've ever heard it. We are nearly out of control. We make accusations the whole way to the restaurant.

Suddenly, in the parking ramp, we run out of energy. We stop shouting. We get out of the car and lock the doors. Both of us are shaking. We take hold of each other's arms for crucial support. The idea that we are on our way to a social event where we will be expected to make conversation and act like normal human beings seems unreal. My throat is sore. We meet our friend at the restaurant and order our dinners.

The nurse practitioner and our primary nurse are waiting for us in Sophia's room when we arrive at the hospital later that night. After my earlier demands over the phone, I am self-conscious, imagining that they're looking at me as if I'm one of those erratic, out-of-control mothers. Maybe I finally am.

We don't get answers to the ultrasound reading that night. There really is a delay, nothing malicious, just a lag of information. It will come through tomorrow.

At home that night, I stay up to pump, though I have never been this tired. I'm surprised I produce any milk at all. I feel empty in so many ways.

The next morning, the nurse practitioner calls. She has conferred with the radiology department and has good news: the increased fluid first noted in the ultrasound is "of no clinical significance." The expected feeling of relief is dulled by exhaustion.

Transition

We arrive for a feeding and find Sophia fussing and scrunched into a ball with her NG tube pulled half-out. This isn't neglect, it's the reality of a busy level two hospital nursery. Each nurse has several charges, and at the moment there are crises to attend to. Sophia is a well baby, just one who needs to learn how to eat dependably.

The neonatologist present at her birth had, early in her hospitalization, told us, "Our goal is to make her into a boring baby." They have succeeded. She's wonderfully dull . . . exquisitely uninteresting.

The latest dreaded eye exam showed that the retinopathy of prematurity is, abruptly, resolving itself.

The heart rate drops are more and more sporadic, occurring most often during feedings, when she's struggling to coordinate the complicated sequence of breathing, sucking, and swallowing.

In fact, there's an annoying sameness to our routine

now. Predictability adds to the stress of the place. Maybe this is what a third trimester feels like. We are preparing for the next stage of this gestation—birth—and the transition to home.

Scott scavenges chairs from another room (there are never enough seats in the nursery; we play an ongoing game of musical chairs), and I throw off my coat. It's fall now. We wash our hands at the sink. When I pick Sophia up, she feels warm and substantial in my arms. She weighs nearly four and a half pounds.

"For months," Scott says, "I thought she belonged in the hospital. Now I think it's time for her to come home."

Freedom

One of the nurses, a vivacious one who is a wonderful contrast to our general weariness, disconnects the apnea monitor, packages Sophia in blankets, and insists we take her for a walk.

Scott is enthused. I am reticent, but I don't argue with what seems to be an exercise designed to make us comfortable caring for our baby beyond the nurses' reassuring reach.

We walk Sophia up and down the hall outside the nursery. We have never been so free and untethered.

Preparations

Although family members have all along suggested that we get started shopping for nursery equipment and clothing, we have purchased nothing. Until now I have been unable to picture Sophia in any environment besides the hospital. At home, the room we said would become a nursery is still a guest room with dingy-gray, nail-marred walls and a queen-sized bed that takes up all but a narrow aisle of walking space.

Now, with neonatologists and nurses all hinting that Sophia may be leaving the hospital within days, Scott takes time off from work to transform the room.

He fills the nail holes and lines the gaps around the window molding with caulk.

He paints the walls a soft, buttery yellow and adds a hand-painted ornamental border and pattern of translucent pink rosebuds. The marathon fix-up puts him in a a good mood. He is a new person.

We shop for nursery essentials—a rocker, rug, bassinet. Our excitement must be a little taste of how normal parents feel as they plan for imminent birth.

The date is set: Sophia will be released tomorrow evening, two days after her due date.

In a rush, Scott puts together the glider and bassinet. He paints the closet while I scrub the floor.

The rug goes down at eleven o'clock.

Bed by midnight.

We don't sleep well. Sophia is coming home.

Homecoming

We tidy our desks and say good-bye to co-workers as if we are leaving for a vacation in a distant location. It is rush hour when we leave the office for the hospital.

Everyone else—as usual—is driving in slow motion. Tonight we're more forgiving. When we pull into the parking ramp, we are beginning to feel jubilant.

The nurses greet us with enthusiasm. While Sophia has dinner of warm breastmilk from a bottle, we pack. There are hugs and well wishes. This is everyone's success. No one is sorry to see us go.

We suddenly find ourselves walking out the door, with Sophia in her father's arms. No one stops us. We keep right on walking down the hall and through the skyway—the ones we have traveled innumerable times during the past four months—to the parking ramp. We're alone with our newborn.

Packed in with rolled towels, Sophia sleeps in the

premie-sized car seat while the green monitor blinks beside her.

The dogs come out to greet us in the yard, as they did the day I first arrived home from the hospital. Keist barks insanely. Both dogs do a thorough sniffing of the baby's head. Scott and I take pictures of each other holding Sophia in the dining room, where we began this journey, grinning like fools.

It is our fourteenth wedding anniversary. While Scott opens the champagne I chilled that morning, I make a celebration dinner, and Sophia sleeps in her new bassinet. We open gifts in the sunroom. My aunt and uncle have sent red and pink roses to mark Sophia's homecoming.

I nurse Sophia, sitting cross-legged on the couch. For the first time since July eleventh, there is nowhere else we should be. We are all together.

A few days later, the notice arrives in the mail, a belated update from the wildlife refuge center. The staff is pleased to report that the baby starling we rescued and delivered to them last summer was nursed to maturity and released.

Sophia Olivia Nielsen Barsuhn

July 11, 1994
6:11 PM
1 pound, 7 ounces
12 1/4 inches long

Scott and Shelly are thrilled to announce the birth and long-awaited homecoming of their daughter Sophia who, having overcome many obstacles (and having reached the top of the cuteness scale), was released from the hospital on November 1, two days after her October 30 due date.

Her arrival was heralded by the barking of dogs and the immeasurable happiness of her parents.

Distance; an Epilogue

Someone told me there is an anesthesic that, instead of putting you to sleep, gives you amnesia. When you wake, you remember nothing of the discomfort you have experienced—as if reliving the ordeal were the painful part and not the original pain itself. Though it seemed unimaginable during the four months of Sophia's hospitalization, time at home following her discharge brought with it a kind of selective amnesia.

We were following a very strict quarantine prescribed by her new pediatrician, trying to keep Sophia's lungs safe from viruses. I set up an office at home and between modem sessions, breastfed, bottlefed, and washed my hands compulsively. Scott worked doubletime at the studio and, in the evenings, rocked, bottlefed, and washed his hands compulsively. It was a busy but quiet winter. I only remember Garrison Keillor's voice reading "The Writer's Almanac" on the radio and the buzz of documents coming through the fax. Though nights of uninterrupted sleep were a luxury of times past, I don't remember Sophia's cries. After the cacophony of the hospital, I was in a kind of cottony bliss.

I stopped having the nightly anxiety dream. We looked at Sophia's early photographs with amazement—was she really that small, that sick? We recounted to each other the story of her birth with veteran bravado. We could afford this newfound objectivity. We were no longer in danger.

Though statistically Sophia was at great risk for developing problems, she now shows few signs of her premature birth. We know that forty days on the ventilator caused damage to her lungs, but that the damage has not, so far, slowed her. We have had a "good outcome," as the nurses used to say. Our daughter can do a jazzy snap of her fingers, say "Ha!" with just the right sardonic emphasis, and—if someone holds her hand—walk with the spread-legged swagger of a ranchhand. She embraces every stuffed toy she encounters with frightening intensity and true passion. Her hair is beginning to curl over her ears. Her gums are no longer a smooth, baby pink. They show the crowns of several strong, white teeth.

Distance from the hospital has given us relief, but we are changed. Priorities have been reshuffled, and our patience with the superficial is gone. Though we understand, we sometimes have a hard time relating to people who don't comprehend that we have been through a crisis and will never be the same. And we have an always-present sense that, at any moment, parents are sitting in hospitals, watching over their sick babies.

Scott does not like to visit the hospital. By avoiding the place, he avoids all that he still remembers but tries very hard not to. But as Sophia grows, we will have to revisit those memories, for she will want to know. "How small was I? What did you think when you first saw me? What did I look like?" We will have to practice words that describe how it really felt to love her and wonder if she would live.

A year after her homecoming, I participated in a mothers' support group meeting. Though I had been invited to attend these meetings while Sophia was a patient, I had never felt strong enough to go.

The women sat around tables pushed together in a U. Some brought strollers and babies. Others, those with infants in the NICU downstairs, came alone. At first talk was upbeat, but then, at the social worker's prompting, a young woman with long brown hair, bangs, and a sweet, childlike voice broke down. The room grew quiet and respectful. She had left the hospital the night before feeling good—her two-month-old baby, born at twenty-seven weeks, was doing well. But when she had called in this morning, she learned that he had pneumonia again. She sobbed. He was finally a fat three-pounder, and she didn't know whether he would pull through this time. Every time there was a light at the end of the tunnel, it went dark again.

The woman beside her, who had been jovial early in the meeting, shared the story of her son—a twenty-four-weeker who had such severe problems that the doctors had one last resort left, then, no more options.

A woman told of going into labor with twenty-three-and-a-half week twins at a family wedding. At the small town hospital emergency room the flustered staff had admitted they didn't know what to do. The team from Minneapolis had arrived by helicopter, and she was airlifted to the city. At delivery the doctor had given the babies, a girl and a boy, a thirty-to-forty percent chance of survival. They were three weeks old now and had already been through PDA and intestinal surgeries, and she had no sense that there would ever be an end to this.

I could only listen with helpless empathy. I could fix nothing.

I shared Sophia's story, feeling self-conscious. Though I had suffered greatly with the uncertainty these women described, though I felt a strong bond with them, I had learned the outcome of our story. I was on the other side now. I remembered how I had felt about mothers who revisited the unit with their babies, the ones the nurses liked me to meet—happy for them, but unsure how they related to me, or how their beautiful strong children—already crawling!—related to the scrawny fetus under the phototherapy light. Sophia was surrounded by monitors. She was so weak the ventilator took all of her breaths. Her ribs showed. She was fighting for her life; she might not be so lucky. I couldn't imagine what tomorrow might be like, let alone imagine the possibility of ever escaping the hospital.

I couldn't predict the conclusion of their stories, but I wanted to tell them that they would surprise themselves with their own strength. That their babies were tougher than anyone could expect. That time passes. That it happens slowly, the coming back together.

Coping for Parents

When people ask how Scott and I survived those four months in the hospital, I have no satisfying answer. I know we were blessed. We had each other. Faith in our daughter's will to live and in her innate strength. Faith in God. Family and friends. High technology. Good insurance. Occasional, miraculous shreds of stamina.

In the face of relentless stress, coping devices seemed to me like weak medicine—as if writing poetry were any consolation when Sophia was so sick! We found, however, that the smallest things helped us hang on.

Celebrate the birth.

Like any new parents, we made announcement calls to close family and friends.

The week after Sophia's birth we published an announcement in the local newspaper.

We designed and printed a card containing Sophia's

vital statistics. Our aim with this announcement card was to let people know that, as difficult as the situation was, we were happy about our daughter's birth. (This was, perhaps, too big a project for us, because the piece didn't get produced until the baby arrived home from the hospital. It finally rolled off the press just in time to become a coming-home announcement.)

Take photographs.

Most of our friends and family wouldn't be able to meet Sophia for months, until she was released from the hospital. We felt cheated out of the joy of introducing our baby to the people we loved. One way we helped connect them to our astounding child was through photographs.

Each time we had a roll of film developed, we ordered duplicate prints. We could afford to be generous with pictures, then, and keep people updated on Sophia's progress.

We found an inexpensive magnet frame and attached it to the refrigerator door to display a picture of our baby. Whenever we received a new batch of photographs, we updated the picture. That photo reminded us that we were now parents.

One practical idea—taking photographs of the flowers and balloons we received—helped us keep track of who sent what. Because we were getting duplicate prints of all photos, we could enclose a copy with the thank you card and still have a photo for Sophia's scrapbook.

Record your baby's amazing gestation.

Although time seemed to be standing still, Sophia was gestating before our eyes. Only when we compared the latest batch of photographs with pictures just weeks old did we realize how quickly she was changing.

We didn't own a video camera, so we borrowed one from a generous friend.

We kept a notebook near the phone. During each call to the hospital we jotted the date and time of the update and wrote down any details reported by the nurse—weight, medications given, problems.

Once Sophia was off the ventilator, we made a cassette tape of her voice and added to the recording every week or so.

Some hospitals provide a special keepsake book or calendar to the parents of premature infants. We received a blank calendar with squares just large enough to write in Sophia's weight for the day plus one other bit of information. We could handle this minor, daily task without feeling overwhelmed by obligation.

If you don't receive something like this, adopt your own calendar from a stationery supply store. Keep it at the hospital and write the day's highlights in each box. Record weights, measurements, and all the firsts—first gavage feeding, first "house" change, first day off the ventilator.

We made an effort—for ourselves—to keep up the calendar, but we also did it for Sophia. Our hope was that someday she would be *well*—big enough and old enough to read the diary of her beginnings. Her pediatrician predicted, "She will never tire of hearing the story."

Keep a journal.

I wrote in a notebook every day—a fatiguing and, at times, painful exercise. I didn't do it for therapy; sometimes it was difficult enough getting through a day without having to relive it in a journal entry. I wrote because there was so much going on, so many important, life-altering events, I didn't trust my memory. I forced myself to chronicle the day in ink. Even on the days when

I thought "I just want to forget everything," I wrote, fearing that I would lose track of vital details. The journal is my only record of how I really felt during those long weeks and of the progress Sophia, in tiny increments, was making.

If you don't write, tape record the highlights of the day. These don't have to be earth-shattering observations, just your impressions and thoughts.

Advocate for your baby.

We found that advocacy is a powerful antidote to powerlessness. We became Sophia's champions.

We took on the role gradually as we gained confidence in our own instincts and once we realized, with great surprise, that the learned doctors and nurses *listened* to us.

Our requests ranged from simple ("She's more comfortable when her legs are wrapped; could we put her in a Snugli?") to significant ("We'd eventually like her to be on breast milk only. Is that a possibility?") We respected the professionals and relied on their experience and advice, but we also learned to honor our own intuition because it was based on an intimate knowledge of our daughter. We spent hours with her every day, and visited seven days a week. Even the most dedicated primary nurses couldn't compete with the hours we logged. No one knew her as we did.

Parent your baby.

The traditional parenting activities—diapering, rocking, singing—may be limited at first. You may need to be creative about what you can offer.

Before Sophia was big enough for even the pre-premie diapers, the nurses showed me how to make tiny ones out of cotton gauze. They sent me home with rolls of the stuff, which I cut into strips and assembled with enthusiasm. At last, I was *doing* something.

Scott designed and created a photo album with hand-lettered captions.

I made a short tape of lullabies from childhood records. They were sappy enough to make me cry while I recorded them, but creating that tape for my daughter to listen to *someday* made me feel hopeful and useful.

Later, when invited by the nurses, we helped with temperature-taking, turning, and diaper-changing. We did what we could do.

Realize that you and your partner will deal with this experience in different ways.

Accepting this simple fact may be all you can do for a while.

For me, it was a big first step, realizing that it was permissible for Scott to be depressed when I was hopeful, or easygoing when I was angry. But it took a long time, and merely reaching the *realization* didn't shelter me—or him—from feelings of hurt, rage, and hopelessness.

Heroic measures—understanding, openness, and forgiveness—were needed, attributes we weren't always capable of providing to each other. Some days we did well. Some days we failed each other. I don't pretend to have answers. I don't even say that we always followed these suggestions. But I think we would have benefited from them.

- For this moment, try to view your circumstance from your partner's perspective. If you can't understand his or her viewpoint, can you accept it?
- Forgive harsh words. This is a crisis situation.
- Find simple ways to nurture each other. Include

tender notes, tokens of affection, embraces, strong cups of coffee, and back massages among your techniques.

• Give each other room—time alone and time off from your usual obligations.

• Talk to each other, but be sensitive; your partner may be talked out.

• Consider accepting help from a social worker, outside counselor, or clergy.

Forgive the people who say stupid things.

There will be all kinds of hurts as people struggle to say the right thing. You will need to prepare yourself, too, for the people who don't struggle at all, but spout the first idiotic thought that comes to mind.

"At least you didn't have to go through *real* labor," a friend said to me soon after Sophia's arrival. The recollection of labor was still vivid in my mind, and I didn't take kindly to this comment. (Apparently my body didn't know that babies other than the full-term variety don't require *bona fide* contractions; it could have saved me significant and lengthy discomfort.)

"Think of all the school lunches the money being spent on your daughter could buy for normal kids." This compassionate observation can be attributed to a former acquaintance of Scott's.

More than one individual admitted that since they assumed Sophia wouldn't make it, they didn't buy a present. I believe these people thought they were being kind, but we didn't want to hear that friends assumed our baby would die.

Besides memorable one-liners, you will probably hear many premie success stories. You may find this encouraging, or you may think, "This is my baby, and he's very sick! I don't care about your cousin's sister-in-law's son!" Other people will feel the need to tell you about the premature babies they've heard about who didn't make it, or who would be "better off" if they hadn't made it.

We found that the ratio of kind words to offensive, insensitive, out-and-out cruel, and shocking ones was heavily weighted toward the latter. So to those who, understandably, couldn't imagine what it must be like to be living in terror and sadness, we closed our sensitive ears and turned instead toward friends who said, "We're praying for you" or "How are you guys holding up?"

Have faith.

I didn't feel strong, but faith in God gave me a place to cower, cry, and, sometimes, rest. I was no inspiring monument to piety. I felt like a child, weak and afraid. "Dear God . . ." That's about as far as I got in my prayers, sometimes. It was all my frantic heart could articulate. "Father, please. . . ." Pleading.

God's gift to us was a recognition of—a faith in—Sophia's strength. From the first she surprised us with her stamina. We knew there was no guarantee that everything would turn out all right, but it was clear that she was doing her best, fighting to live.

We had faith, too, in medical technology, but we never turned over our wholehearted trust. There were too many variables, too many things that could go wrong. We had seen things go suddenly awry.

We were fortunate to have doctors who appeared to understand the limits of their skills. How would they know when interventions were hopeless or purely cruel? The neonatologist who had attended Sophia's birth answered this question with what struck me as profound wisdom. "We let the babies tell us."

Rely on friends.

"Please let us know if there's anything we can do—"

We heard this phrase often; people wanted to help but had no idea what was needed.

We had lots of needs, but we weren't comfortable asking for help. I wish we'd thought to have a trusted friend coordinate volunteer efforts. We could have confided our needs, and he or she could have spread the word:

"The lawn needs mowing."

"Weeds are taking over the vegetable garden."

"The house hasn't been vacuumed in three weeks."

"The dogs need to be let out twice a day while we're at the hospital."

"We're too tired to cook. We'll eat anything you bring—sandwiches, pizza, or a casserole."

Establish rituals.

A hospitalized infant means that, overnight, all of your old routines disappear, to be replaced by chaos.

For sanity, almost by instinct, we created a new set of rituals to depend on. They added routine and security to the week.

The pasta dinner, a weekly event, was carved in stone. You don't have to be a good cook to pull this off. This is an improvised, very easy recipe for a filling dinner.

COMFORT PASTA WITH GARLIC

1/2 - 1 lb dried pasta (spaghetti, spaghettini, or fettuccine)
Olive oil (about 1/4 cup)
Garlic (5-7 cloves, more or less, depending on your taste)

Fresh parsley (Italian flat leaf or conventional - about 12 branches)
Parmesan cheese, finely grated (about 1/2 cup)

1. Heat a big pot of water to boiling.

2. Drop the pasta into the boiling water and stir to make sure the pieces don't stick.

3. Pour the olive oil into a large skillet and heat on medium-high.

4. Mince the garlic and add to the oil, turning down the heat a bit so it cooks nicely but doesn't brown.

5. Meanwhile, chop the leaves of the parsley and set aside.

6. When the pasta is *al dente*, drain and add to the skillet, turning the spaghetti to coat with the garlic-oil mixture.

7. Stir in the parsley and parmesan cheese. Mix thoroughly and serve.

Serve with hot bread and a salad.

NOTE: Speed and ease were my two primary goals. To avoid dealing with clingy garlic peelings, get a clove out of its skin in this way:

Place the garlic clove on a cutting board. Lay a large knife over the clove, blade flat. Give the blade a good whack with your fist or the heel of your hand. The clove will crack and the skin of the garlic should now peel off easily.

SIMPLE GREEN SALAD

Lettuce greens
(if you can find it and afford it, buy a pre-washed lettuce mixture)
Raw vegetables (as desired)

1. Tear washed and dried greens into a large bowl. Add chopped vegetables.

2. In a lidded jar, combine the vinaigrette ingredients:

   2 T. red wine vinegar or good balsamic vinegar
   3 T. olive oil

3. Shake well. Pour as much as you like over the greens and toss well. Add salt and fresh ground pepper to taste.

Scott's second favorite new survival ritual involved getting up early Saturday mornings, buying cream cheese and bags of bagels at a local shop, and driving alone to the hospital. He would arrive just as the morning shift was coming out of "report," and distribute treats to everyone.

The nurses loved this. I slept in and Scott got some time alone with Sophia.

I most looked forward to a weekly Sunday morning walk to a neighborhood coffee shop. Our destination was a substantial distance away. The walk there required an outlay of energy, which probably helped relieve stress. We had a moment to pretend we had a normal life. We had time to talk. We had time together to fantasize about our daughter's homecoming.

Light a candle.

Evenings after work and always during our Saturday night dinners, we lit a large, scented candle. Somehow, that light in the dark of the living room made us more able to bear Sophia's absence.

Play music.

Our friend's gift of a cassette tape—Enya's "Shepherd Moons"—was intended for Sophia, but it became our theme music. (This was after the first shock of Sophia's birth, when we were again able to listen to music.) We played it driving to the hospital; we played it driving home again. For months we listened to nothing else. We were soothed by the repetition. The music was gentle and asked nothing of us.

When Sophia finally came home, we returned the gift to her. Each night we rocked her to the lyrics we had memorized for solace.

Treat yourself kindly.

People were always advising us to see movies, go to dinner, relax, enjoy ourselves. We found it difficult, especially at first, to have a good time when we were so worried about Sophia.

So we compromised. Our refuge was coffee. I have never, before or since, drunk as much coffee as I did that summer and fall. We stopped for coffee-to-go nearly every morning. We bought coffees at a cart in the hospital. During our evening visits to Sophia we sometimes walked for coffee at the fast food restaurant in the adjoining hospital. This is only an example of how a small treat—something to look forward to—helped us cope.

Talk to others who know.

If you would like to talk to someone who has survived a premature birth, the unit social worker will connect you with an appropriate resource. This may mean getting in touch with graduate families or attending support group sessions.

We talked with fellow parents but we also depended on the legion of nurses who assisted with Sophia's out-of-uterus gestation. They helped us survive by letting us talk and by conveying their knowledge in a caring way.

I will always be grateful to them for their expertise and compassion.

Terms

ABRUPTION - The early separation of the placenta from the uterine wall.

ALVEOLI - Tiny air sacs in the lungs.

AMPICILLIN - An antibiotic used to treat infection.

ANEMIA - A condition resulting from too few red blood cells in the blood. Because red blood cells deliver oxygen, a shortage of these cells can prevent sufficient oxygen from reaching the body's cells and tissues. Note: many newborns experience anemia; the nurses and doctors caring for preterm infants watch to be certain that this condition is not the result of blood loss or illness.

APNEA - An incident in which the baby stops breathing for more than fifteen or twenty seconds.

BAGGING - Manually pressing air and/or oxygen in and out of the lungs, usually by covering the nose and mouth with a mask and using a hand-operated ventilator pump.

BILIRUBIN - The substance created when red blood cells break down. If too much bilirubin accumulates in the blood, the baby becomes jaundiced. In very rare cases, damage to the central nervous system can result if the levels rise very high.

BILILIGHT - The phototherapy light used to treat the excess of bilirubin in the blood. It helps the baby's organs change this waste product (created during red cell breakdown) into a harmless substance that can be excreted from the body through urine and stools.

BETAMETHASONE - A type of steroid injected into the mother before a preterm baby's birth to speed the development of the lungs.

BLOOD GAS - A blood test performed to analyze the baby's blood for current levels of oxygen, carbon dioxide, and acid. This test monitors how well the lungs are functioning in combination with other support (ventilator or drugs).

BRADYCARDIA - A lower than normal heart rate—fewer than 80 beats per minute.

BRAIN BLEED - Hemorrhaging into the brain.

CAFFEINE - A stimulant sometimes prescribed to help reduce apnea spells.

CC - A unit of measure, short for cubic centimeter. Thirty ccs equal one ounce.

CARDIOPULMONARY RESUSCITATION (CPR) - Resuscitation techniques used when an infant's breathing or heartbeat has stopped or slowed.

CATHETER - A thin tube inserted into the body to administer fluids or drain fluids.

CENTRAL LINE - An intravenous line threaded through the vein and positioned close to the heart.

CEREBRAL PALSY - A condition describing any abnormal muscle function or difficulty with coordinated movement, caused by a brain injury.

CHRONIC LUNG DISEASE (CLD) - (also broncho-pulmonary dysplasia or BDP) The damage to the lungs caused by oxygen and/or ventilator pressures. This disease is often seen in infants suffering from respiratory distress syndrome who spend a long period of time on a ventilator.

CLINICAL NURSE SPECIALIST - An advance practice nurse who has a master's degree in nursing or public health and whose responsibilities often focus more on education and research than direct patient care.

CONTINUOUS POSITIVE AIRWAY PRESSURE (CPAP) - A method of delivering pressurized air or oxygen through a face mask, cannula, or endotracheal tube to keep the baby's lungs partially expanded after he or she exhales.

CORRECTED GESTATIONAL AGE - (also adjusted age) The age of a preterm baby based on his or her due date (instead of his or her actual birth date). For example, a baby who was born five months ago but who was four months early is one month old, counting from his or her original due date.

DECADRON - The trade name for dexamethasone, a steroid.

DESATURATION (DESAT) - A decrease in the oxygen content in the blood. Acceptable levels are based on the infant's health and condition.

DIURETIC - A drug that helps the body excrete excess fluids that have accumulated in the lungs and body. These excess fluids are passed through urine.

EDEMA - Excess fluid resulting in puffiness or swelling.

EMERGENCY MEDICAL TECHNICIAN (EMT) - An individual with special medical training to handle emergency transports to hospitals.

ENDOTRACHEAL TUBE (ET) - A tube inserted into the baby's airway to allow delivery of air and/or oxygen to the lungs via the ventilator.

EXTUBATION - The removal of the ET tube.

FETUS - The term used to describe a baby from the twelfth week of pregnancy until the date of delivery.

FULL-TERM - A baby born between the thirty-eighth and forty-second weeks of gestation.

GAVAGE FEEDING - A feeding through a tube that has been inserted through the nose or mouth and into the stomach.

GRAM - A unit of measure. Twenty-eight grams equal one ounce.

HEEL STICK - The pricking of the heel to obtain a blood sample.

HEMATOCRIT - The percentage of red blood cells to plasma (body fluid) in the blood.

HUMAN MILK FORTIFIER (HMF) - A powdered substance added to breast milk to increase its nutritive and caloric value.

HYDROCEPHALUS - The accumulation of spinal fluid in the ventricles (chambers) of the brain.

INCUBATOR - (also isolette or house) The plastic "box" or environment that insulates babies from heat and fluid loss. It enables a preterm baby's temperature, oxygen, and humidity to be controlled, allows access and observation to medical personnel, and minimizes the environmental stresses of sounds and lights.

INTUBATION - The insertion of the endotracheal tube into the windpipe.

IV - A tube or needle inserted into the vein for the administering of fluids (nutrition or medication).

JAUNDICE - A condition that results in the yellowing of the skin and whites of the eyes, caused by an excess amount of bilirubin—a waste product—in the blood.

LASIX - A diuretic that pulls excess fluid from the lungs, allowing injured lungs to work better.

MAGNESIUM SULFATE - A closely monitored drug used to stop pre-term labor by relaxing body muscles.

NASAL CANNULA - Flexible tubing with prongs that fit into the nostrils for the delivery of oxygen or air.

NASO-GASTRIC TUBE (NG) - A thin, flexible tube inserted through the nose into the stomach. Feedings administered through this tube are commonly called gavage feedings.

NEBULIZER - A device used to deliver vaporized medication to the nose and lungs.

NECROTIZING ENTERCOLITIS (NEC) - A disease of the intestinal tract caused by many factors and not thoroughly understood. It is more common in preterm babies than full-term infants.

NEONATOLOGIST - A physician whose specialty extends from pediatrics to the care of critically ill newborns, usually from birth to day twenty-eight of life. A neonatologist can often be involved as the primary care provider beyond this period for newborns with complicated initial health histories.

NURSE PRACTITIONER - A registered nurse with advanced technical and assessment skills who (under physician supervision) performs many of the functions assigned to physicians including medication prescription, invasive procedures such as intubation, and laboratory interpretation.

PATENT (OPEN) DUCTUS ARTERIOSUS (PDA) - A fetal blood vessel connecting the aorta and the pulmonary artery which in healthy, full-term babies usually closes within hours of birth.

PERCUSSION, SUCTIONING, AND VIBRATION - A treatment to loosen and remove the mucus that accumulates in the lungs. Vibration and thumping on the chest are followed by the vacuuming—or suctioning—of the mucus through a tube.

PERINATOLOGIST - A physician who specializes in the management of high-risk pregnancies.

PHOTOTHERAPY - A method of using specific light spectrums to treat infants who have excess bilirubin in the blood by creating chemical changes through the skin.

POSTPARTUM - A period of time after the birth.

PRETERM - A baby born before the thirty-eighth week of gestation.

PULMONARY EDEMA - The accumulation of fluid in the lungs.

PULSE OXIMETER - A machine that constantly tracks the oxygen content of the blood.

REGISTERED NURSE - An individual educated to perform a variety of tasks to facilitate recovery from illness and assess patient responses to prescribed therapies. A registered nurse is licensed to work after satisfying the educational requirements defined by the state board of nursing. An R.N. must also meet the educational and performance requirements of the employing institution.

RESPIRATORY DISTRESS SYNDROME (RDS) - (also hyaline membrane disease - HMD) A condition common in premature babies, resulting from the lack of sufficient surfactant in the lungs. RDS causes breathing difficulties.

RESPIRATORY THERAPIST (RT) - A specially trained technician who administers inhaled medications, adjusts ventilator settings, and sets up respiratory equipment.

RETINOPATHY OF PREMATURITY - A disease that can affect the retina of premature infants.

STIM - Short for stimulation. If a nurse says, "I had to stim the baby," it means she had to gently wiggle his leg or stroke him to bring him out of an apnea spell.

SURFACTANT - The lubricating substance that coats the alveoli and keeps the lungs from collapsing.

SURVANTA - The trade name for synthetic surfactant replacement given to newborn premature babies with respiratory distress syndrome.

TACHYCARDIA - A higher than normal heart rate.

TACHYPNEA - A higher than normal breathing rate.

TERBUTALINE - A drug used to relax the uterus and stop pre-term labor.

THEOPHYLLINE - An oral medication given to help reduce apnea.

VENTILATOR - (also respirator) A machine that helps the baby breathe—or artificially breathes for the baby. It supplies oxygen and pressure as needed to support the work of the lungs.

Bibliography and Resources

When you look for books about prematurity, note the date of publication and whether the book has been recently updated. The field of neonatology is changing rapidly. Older volumes may not have the latest, most accurate technical data; even a year or two can make a difference. These books may still contain valuable information. If you have questions about anything you read, consult your baby's caregivers.

Some of the books listed are out of print, but may be found in the library.

PREMATURITY AND RELATED TOPICS

Pamphlets—

Many free, well-written pamphlets about prematurity are

distributed by formula manufacturers. They are usually displayed in parent rooms or lobbies. In addition, the following pamphlets may be helpful.

"Understanding My Signals; Help for Parents of Premature Infants"
Brenda Hussey, M.A., MPH
VORT Corporation
P.O. Box 60132
Palo Alto, CA 94306

Available from Centering Corporation, 1531 North Saddle Creek Road, Omaha, NE 68104, (402) 553-1200:

"Baby Talk"
Dale Hatcher and Kathy Lehman

"Daddy: NICU"
(A number of fathers talk about their NICU babies)

"No Bigger Than My Teddy Bear"
Valerie Pankow

Available from A Place To Remember, c/o deRuyter-Nelson Publications, Inc., 1885 University Avenue, Suite 110, St. Paul, MN 55104, 1-800-631-0973:

"A Fragile Beginning: Parenting Your Early Baby"

"Katie's Premature Brother"
Elizabeth Hawkins-Walsh

"Our New Baby Needs Special Help"
Gail Klayman with illustrations by Shari Borum

Books—

Kangaroo Care
Susan Ludington-Hoe
Bantam Books

My NICU Baby Book
Edited by Joy Johnson
A fill-in-the-blank baby book especially for premature infants, available from A Place To Remember, c/o deRuyter-Nelson Publications, Inc., 1885 University Avenue, Suite 110, St. Paul, MN 55104, 1-800-631-0973

Parenting Your Premature Baby
Janine Jason and Antonia Van Der Meer
Henry Holt & Company

Premature Babies: A Different Beginning
W. A. H. Sammons and J. M. Lewis
The C.V. Mosby Company

The Premature Baby Book
Helen Harrison with Ann Kositsky, RN
St. Martin's Press

Your Premature Baby
Frank P. Manginello, MD and
Teresa Foy DiGeronimo, MED
John Wiley and Sons, Inc.

Other Resources—

Parent Care, Inc. is an international not-for-profit organization offering a quarterly newsletter—*News Brief*—publications, videos, help forming and maintaining local support groups, and more, for the parents of premature and high-risk infants. For membership information, contact:
Parent Care, Inc.
9041 Colgate Street
Indianapolis, IN 46268-1210
(317) 872-9913

BREASTFEEDING

Pamphlets—

"Breastfeeding Your Premature or Special Care Baby; A Practical Guide for Nursing the Tiny Baby"
Marsha Walker, RN, BS, IBCLC
Lactation Associates
254 Conant Road
Weston, MA 02193-1756

"A Gift of Love; Your Guide to Breast Feeding"
American Academy of Pediatrics
Publications Department
P.O. Box 927
Elk Grove Village, IL 60009-0927
(847) 228-5005

"Nursing Your Premature Baby"
Sarah Coulter Danner, CPNP, CNM
and Edward R. Cerutti, MD
Childbirth Graphics
P.O. Box 21207
Waco, TX 76702-1207
800-299-3366

Books—

All are offered by La Leche League International. To order, call (847) 519-9585.

Breastfeeding Pure and Simple
Gwen Gotsch

The Breastfeeding Answer Book
Nancy Mohrbacher and Julie Stock

Mothering Multiples; Breastfeeding and Caring for Twins
Karen Gromada

The Womanly Art of Breastfeeding

Support Groups—

To find a La Leche League support group in your area, contact:
La Leche League International
1400 North Meacham Road
Schaumburg, IL 60173-4840
1-800-LA-LECHE

To locate a lactation consultant, contact:
International Lactation Consultant Association
200 North Michigan Avenue
Chicago, IL 60601
(312) 541-1710

Pump Supplies and Rentals—

To receive information regarding Ameda-Egnell rental supplies and breast pumps in your area, or to locate a lactation consultant, contact the customer service department of Ameda-Egnell Corporation at 1-800-323-8750 (708-639-2900/IL).
Ameda-Egnell Corporation
765 Industrial Drive
Cary, IL 60013

For information on renting Medela breast pumps in your area and finding breastfeeding consultants, contact the Breastfeeding National Network at 1-800-835-5968.
c/o Medela, Inc.
P.O. Box 660
McHenry, IL 60051

For More Information—

An excellent and thorough bibliography and resource list, including parent support groups, associations, periodicals, and organizations, appears in *The Premature Baby Book* by Helen Harrison.

The La Leche League offers a research service called the Breastfeeding Reference and Data Base. Staff members will research topics you request and send copies of articles. They have access to more than 10,000 full length articles from professional journals, and there is a category for premature infants. For information on a topic, call (847) 519-7730.

The fee for this service is $25 for the first fifteen minutes, and $15 for each additional 15 minutes. Cost is determined by the time required to discuss, retrieve, and prepare information.